Dr. Micha

CW01509554

# The Little

# QUANTUM
# TEMPLE

## Self Healing with
## modern Physics

This book is published
by the author himself

**Bibliographical Information of the Deutsche Nationalbibliothek**
This publication is listed in the Deutsche Nationalbibliographie of the
Deutsche Nationalbibliothek; detailed bibliographical information
can be accessed under http: //dnb.d-nb.de

This book is a guide for self-healing and for the development of ones
own consciousness. This method can only be used in appropriate
self-care. The book offers no alternative for professional treatement
of severe illnesses and it should not stop you from seeking
conventional medical advice.

Original edition in German:
© 2011 Scorpio Verlag GmbH & Co. KG, Berlin München


© 2014 Michael König
Printing and Production: BoD – Books on Demand
ISBN: 978-3-7357-1091-8


www.drmichaelkoenig.de

For Daniel

# CONTENT

# A Glimpse into the Quantum Temple

Many people nowadays are no longer merely concerned with satisfying their material needs - they also view their life as a spiritual adventure. Self-discovery, a sense of purpose and further spiritual further development – transformation - have become fundamental requirements for them. In biophysical terms, spiritual transformation means fanning the flames of the human energy system.

Individual people like you and me are the architects of their own fortune – happiness and love incessantly surround us as divine primal substances in the form of an omnipresent quantum ocean and are just waiting to resonate with each living being. By means of the transformation methods presented and described in the chapters of this book, each individual person can make their own personal flame of happiness burn brightly.

Based upon the findings of quantum and biophysics, it is today possible to present and practise methods of personal development and spiritual transformation, detached from the ideological "make-up". Today, the entity of mind, body and soul is also affirmed through natural science: it is intended that the methods and exercises presented here should help to mobilise the happiness potential for this entity.

Through their application, everyone can learn to acknowledge, know and love themselves and others with greater intensity. They help us to switch on our biophoton "lamps" in order to flood all rooms and recesses of our soul with comforting warmth and light. The only thing that we need for this is a little peace and time for ourselves.

## ABOUT QUANTA AND PHOTONS – A BRIEF DEFINITION OF THE TERMS

Quantum healing is "in" – natural science and spirituality are celebrating their "marriage"! But what does "quantum" actually mean? What are "quanta" indeed?

Everything that we are able to see and touch is comprised of atoms and molecules. These are constructed from elementary particles such as protons, neutrons and electrons, which exchange photons and neutrinos between each other (I describe neutrinos more generally as ETA particles; please also refer to page 78f). In my Ancient Word Theory, I revealed how photons and electrons can be described by means of combinations - or rather, swirls - of eta-particles.

In physics, all such elementary particles are generally described as quanta. A quantum (in Latin, "quantum" = how much, how large) contains a certain portion of energy in the form of mass, rotation, movement and information.

Where do photons come from? Physicists have

discovered that photons are largely emitted from - and received by - electrons. They exist in every atom and molecule of our body. Several theories are based upon the assumption that electrons have a kind of memory. In their inner space-time, they store encounters and exchange processes with other quanta in the form of patterns of light. These are certain arrangements of photons. By means of their inner patterns of light, the electrons determine the energy and information of the photons that they emit, which they exchange with other electrons. As a logical consequence, processes - such as emotions and thoughts and other states of consciousness - can be described through the nature of the quantum fields in our body. Not only does the two-way arrangement of atoms and molecules to one another, as well as their energy status, determine the outer form and design of our body, but also the quality of our consciousness. At the same time a key role is played by the internal order – the coherence – of the quantum fields.

We now know that vitality, quality of life and consciousness are dependent upon the amount and quality of the photons in our body. Photons are small portions of electromagnetic radiation - these equally include the photons of visible light radiation, which we are able to see with our eyes, and the more energy-rich UV photons, as well as very high energy x-ray and gamma quanta, and the lower energy photons of heat radiation and longer-wave radiation.

The photons in biological organisms are also known as biophotons. They move back and forth between our body's atoms and molecules and, in doing so, guide the metabolic processes in our body's cells. However, their energy can also be stored in atoms and molecules. When this occurs in our cells, the electrons in the atomic shells can become detached and loose as a result. Bioplasma is thus created in our body – a mix comprising detached, negatively charged electrons and positively charged residual atoms.

## OUR BODY IS THE QUANTUM TEMPLE

It comprises billions of cells, for example cells from skin, muscles, bones, blood and nerves. These form our organs and body structures: head, upper and lower body, arms and legs, hands and feet. The photons play a very important role in the functioning of our organism and in the whole system working together smoothly. In this way, billions upon billions of photons are continuously exchanged in and among our cells in order to control metabolic and growth processes.

In each cell, the substances that are supplied from outside, such as sugar, fat and protein, are further processed in order to turn them into specific protein molecules, which for example work like small robots to - in turn - create other molecules. In our bodies there prevails a continuous flowing and joining together of different substances, all controlled by a highly coherent photon field.

This all works without us consciously controlling it. Our body alerts us that it needs fluid and nourishment or that it wants to eliminate something. So far so good. However: going way beyond these basic vegetative functions is the relationship that we have with our body. But who - or what - are we?

Well, we are our body and we are that in which we feel within our body – pleasure or pain, love or irritation, sadness or anger, or – happiness.

We now know that certain chemical conditions are connected with our feelings. If we say, "I am mad" (the German language is more precise here, stating "I am sour") then that is a description of a feeling of irritation and anger, but we are sour in chemical terms, in the sense of an excess of sourness – there is a lack of electrons. If we are joyful and happy, part of a certain molecule is present in our body – endorphins. All of these molecules also correspond with certain photon fields in our bodies. They generate free electrons and vice versa.

If we are happy, then a sufficient amount of free electrons are present in our body. They ensure for a powerfully regulated photon field in our cells. It is as though somebody has lit a comforting, glowing candle within us, or even switched on the floodlight – our body then possesses a high concentration of biophotons. If, at the same time, the photons are highly ordered or - in other words - coherent, they remain bundled together like a laser beam for a longer period. Our state of happiness then remains within us for a longer period. However, if this degree of order within the photon field is not very high, then many photons are incoherent. As a consequence, the happiness is merely a flash in the pan and not something long-lasting. The photons then become scattered and dissipate like the beam of light from an ordinary torch.

If we are unhappy or angry, then there is a lack of electrons in our body. The electrons are those quanta that establish the photon fields within our body. If there is a lack of electrons, it literally becomes darker within us; dark feelings mean the absence of light, a weak photon field.

If we wish to forge our happiness, then we also need a great deal of coherent photons – this creates order and harmony and a high concentration of biophotons.

## DEVELOPING A HIGHER LEVEL OF CONSCIOUSNESS

A weak photon field goes hand in hand with a state of unconsciousness. If we are unaware of something, we do not have the possibility to reflect upon our feelings. Our feelings then dictate to us what we must and must not do. Whether we are currently happy is not dependent upon our decision, but rather upon external factors. It is as if we would live in a house where somebody would indiscriminately switch a light on or off. In the extreme situation, we would swing between feelings of ecstatic joy one minute followed by deep despair the next.

A small child cries or screams the very instant that it is not happy about something. A moment later it can laugh again when the fun barometer has exceeded a certain threshold level. The child is still very unaware and its emotions are dependent upon its parents. Many people do not overcome this dependence by means of personal maturity and development of consciousness. Thus, their relationships to others are often marked by expectations – the breeding ground for possessiveness and jealousy.

We are actually all designed to be able to experience an excess of happiness and love, generated from within ourselves, without mental and emotional dependence upon other people. Such dependence reduces the quality of life and the ability to experience deep fulfilment. The key to liberation is to develop consciousness in order to dissolve old patterns of thought and to bid farewell to conditioning and behaviour that inhibit happiness.

Unaware of better alternatives, during the course of their lives most people start to suppress their feelings in order to take mental control of their life by means of their intellect and thoughts. However, the snag with this is that not only do they cut themselves off from possible flows of happiness, but they are singlely occupied with controlling everything within their thoughts.


## THE POWER OF OUR THOUGHTS

Thoughts correspond with photons. These have a higher frequency than the photon fields of emotions and, as a result, thoughts are able to dominate emotions. And when we think that we are thinking, then it is our electrons that are thinking. Once the electrons have got used to thinking, then they do it unswervingly and incessantly. Our thinking is also insistent. Thought processes - and generally all mental processes - can be described by photon fields that are exchanged with the electrons and molecules in our brain.

The power of thought should not be underestimated. It is through our thoughts that we create the environment in which we live – indeed, it is through our thoughts that we manifest our reality. Everything that we humans have created - whether works of art, tools or machines
– are the products of our thoughts manifested in the form of material. They hold considerable creative powers. Through our thoughts, we establish and find reason for our world; we collect and order experiences; we reflect and analyse.

If we consciously decide to take a life-affirming, positive attitude and give priority to positive thoughts, then we are optimistic. We are also then sufficiently creative to consistently create situations in which we experience something that makes us happy and that provides pleasure for ourselves and for others. This is already a good prerequisite for something even better – the state of pure consciousness without thought, with which we will later concern ourselves in more detail.

Our thoughts are often linked with our emotions. Or the thoughts are so dominant that we often don't notice what it is that we feel. Our thoughts spare our emotions from oscillating too strongly, but the intensity of our ability to feel is reduced as a result.

Most so-called adults live in a state of permanent control through the intellect. Intellect builds upon knowledge and experience. However, it also excludes new experiences and the ability to be adventurous.

Thoughts crystallise into mental attitudes: outlooks, philosophy of life, dogmas, convictions, knowledge... Ideas can become ideologies that have the inherent will to manifest themselves. If we are obsessed by certain ideas, then we become dogmatic and self-opinionated. If we handle our intellectual powers in an unconscious way, we become easy to manipulate.

As positive as they may be, thoughts do not produce endorphins or "happiness hormones". The frequency of the thought photons is not yet sufficient for this. Thinking limits people to within themselves. As a general rule, we are isolated from other people through our own thoughts. In order to share our thoughts with other people, we have to communicate.

However, between some people – especially when they are familiar with each other - there is such a thing as telepathy; they often have the same thoughts at the same time. Telepathy is not imaginary, but rather the interaction between two photon fields. Such a process no longer seems so rare nowadays – people are no longer surprised by how mobile phones, radio and television can connect wirelessly, yet there remain sceptics about telepathy.

Is that really all that we are? The body, memories, expectations, experiences, feelings, a flow of thoughts, thought constructions andknowledge?

## HAPPINESS THAT GOES BEYOND THOUGHTS AND FEELINGS

We are capable of much more than thinking and feeling. If we learn to plunge into a state that is void of thoughts and feelings, then we experience ourselves as pure consciousness. We are happy in this state, and the meditators and mystics throughout time have always recognised that consciousness is always being in the present - now. A powerful effervescence which we are able to discover between our thoughts.

Pure consciousness comprises photons of the highest frequency. They penetrate everything, they are everywhere and they are free. Nothing can hinder them or hold them back. If a photon field from our body meets with this consciousness photon, what we experience is unadulterated happiness – a powerful and vital flow of energy within us. This happiness is then who we are. Meditation is a path to the know-how that this state of happiness is manifested within us and is growing in stability – and this happiness is limitless.

We encounter ourselves - and all of mankind - with love, for happiness Is love. We decide for ourselves whether or not we wish to surrender to certain thought processes. We are no longer the slaves of our thoughts, but rather our intellect becomes a valuable tool that we use when want to and when we need to. And always, if we take a break in our thoughts, then we are in a state of pure consciousness, and a stream of happiness from biophotons floods through our body - flowing from the tops of our heads through to the soles of our feet like a waterfall. Our mind, body and soul become a light-flooded quantum temple.

And if we allow this stream of happiness to continue to grow, then we fan a powerful flame of light made of biophotons, which illuminates us. This is our true nature – a glittering firework of love and happiness. Is that what you want? This is what this booklet is all about. Give it some serious thought. You can still put it aside. There is no going back for anyone who reads to the next line.

✻  ✻  ✻  ✻  ✻  ✻  ✻

In order to fan these flames of happiness, it is necessary to take various transformation steps that are applied to the physical, as well as the spiritual and intellectual levels. In order to reach this goal, it wouldn't make sense to merely undergo certain physical exercises or breathing exercises, to only practise meditation in silence or just to pray. We need a little of everything: the right mixture. For this reason we will turn our attention to the different aspects of a transformation process.

## THE "STUMBLING BLOCK" ON THE PATH TO PURE CONSCIOUSNESS

What is actually preventing us from being able to take up this wonderful state immediately? Unpleasent experiences lead to a disharmonious exchange of photons among our body's electrons. As a result, the concentration of the biophoton fields in our body is reduced. Traumatic experiences lead to blockages, to disturbances of the free flow of energy within our body's own biophoton fields. It loses its coherence, focus and order. We thereby lose vitality in the form of biophotons. The ability to perform and the zest for life becomes less and we become more prone to sickness.

Through experiences that are suppressed rather than being consciously treated, it is inevitable that – during the course of a lifetime – there occur all kinds of mindsets and conditioning, which could impair an individual's quality of life. Each experience, whether pleasant or unpleasant, is imprinted upon the union of our mind, body and soul by means of an exchange of energy and information – through the use of photons.

Every single one of our experiences is stored in our electrons. Also existing within us are photon fields that are more or less energetically and informally restricted to an area of the body, which has been affected by a traumatic experience, from the rest of the body. We perceive such photon fields in the form of anxiety. If we have the courage to face our fears, we are able to consciously process these traumatic experiences and dissipate the associated pain and fields of interference.

## YOU HAVE TO FACE YOUR ANXIETIES

The cycle of the conscious processing of a trauma comprises the memory of the event and the transformation of disharmonious photon fields into a harmonious one. It is precisely this that is the transformation. With every trauma, which we have consciously processed, we reflect the experience and dissolve the associated negative emotional and mental conditioning. Each transformation step thus leads to a heightening of our biophoton concentration and therewith, to an increase in our vitality and zest for life.

It is also a learning process – we want to get to know ourselves, through attentiveness, through the close observation of our pain, feelings and thoughts. We simply want to be here, where we currently are, and all that matters is to always live in the moment – the present. Precisely here and now is where we will find that which makes us happy – not yesterday, which we perhaps mourn, and also not tomorrow, upon which we perhaps project hopes of some kind. Happiness is not waiting for us... it is always there, within us – we are this happiness. This happiness spreads within us when all of our agitation and all of our thoughts have evaporated.

## METHODS FOR TRANSFORMATION

The following will introduce effective methods with which we can increase the biophoton concentration in our bodies and which will help us to adopt the position of an impartial observer in the face of our feelings and thoughts. As a result, we are able to reach a higher state of con-sciousness so that happiness is able to develop within us.

Since my youth I have practised several of these methods myself and developed them further in the mid 1980's as I began to communicate them to other people in the form of spiritual workshops.

They are partially derived from traditional methods, which helped me in my own transformation. I carefully tailored them for the "modern" western civilisation. I have also introduced some methods myself because I have experienced them as being particularly effective, the method of shaking, for example. Over the course of the past year, several have been further refined or were added at a later date. What's new are my quantum meditations, which are introduced for the first time in chapters 3 and 4, as well as the "one-point method" and "zero-point method" of quantum healing, which work more simply and effectively than the "two-point method" presented by other authors.

Most of the transformation methods described in this book – irrespective of whether body-oriented exercises, breathing exercises or meditations – may be practised alone, in pairs or in a group. Of course, it is more fun with more people. At the same time, the exchange of experiences is also important. Naturally it is not about enjoyable companionability, but rather we want to receive a deep access to ourselves, and the spiritual transformation demands our complete attention.

Let's seek a place in which we will not be disturbed or distracted. It should be a room with a clear atmosphere.

# 1. BREATHING EXERCISES

## ABOUT THE BREATHING

Breathing plays a very important role in our transformation, i.e. in the conversion and increase of our electromagnetic energy. Hardly any function of our body is as connected with vitality as breathing. Without breathing, our body would cease to function very quickly.

Have we not all tried as children who can hold their breath the longest? With a little practice we may have been able to hold our breath for a brief minute, but then the reflex overcame us and we were forced to open our mouths and take some violent deep breaths. Trained extreme sportsmen, namely apnea-divers, manage to hold their breath longer than ten minutes and progress to water depths of more than four hundred feet without breathing equipment.

Some Sadhus in India are said to have managed to go for even longer periods of time than that without breathing. Some of them let themselves be buried underground. They probably fall into a state of body stiffness, from which they evolve again when they are brought back to light. The fact that certain animal species can fall into a similar state for longer time spans, the startle rigidity, has already been scientifically proven.

The majority of people breathe mostly unconsciously and give no attention to this process. This is not surprising, because breathing is controlled by the autonomic nervous system, like the heartbeat and it doesn't require a conscious act of will, as a purposeful movement would. Nevertheless, it is possible for us, to control the function of inhalation and exhalation deliberately and this is, as we shall see below, a good thing.

It is still of widespread opinion that breathing essentially serves only to supply the body with oxygen during inhalation and for excreting carbon dioxide during exhalation. This of course is true, but besides that through the molecular metabolism, the gas exchange, we also take in bioplasma while breathing (as already described: electromagnetic energy in the form of photons) into our body.

We know this as fresh air. Any doctor will give a pale couch potato the advice: „Go out more in the fresh air. It will do you good!" But what is so fresh about it? I could set up an oxygen bottle in an unheated appartment with the windows closed and replace as much oxygen as I consume through my breathing to keep the oxygen content of the air constant. In addition, I would have to remove the carbon dioxide with a suitable machine. Similar to what the astronauts do in their space capsules. Then of course, I would surely have plenty of „fresh air" as well.

But this is far from being identical with the fresh air that can be found outside under the open sky. There it is in fact enriched with photons which are constantly exchanged beween the air molecules and thereby cause a plasma state (energetically animated gas state): the bioplasma. If we look carefully at deciduous trees at dusk after a nice summer day, we can observe the shimmering and flickering of biophotons with which the leaves of the trees have charged themselves during the day.

Outdoors, photons with low and high energy portions are present because the sun in particular continuously enriches the molecules of the atmosphere with photons. This is light food that our body needs and we take it in by breathing. Already in the ancient cultures this fact was known and only named differently – the Indians, for example, called it Prana. This is a term for the same form of energy, of which we know today as the photons which are stored in the form of bioplasma in the air.

*Breathing as a way to transformation*

Therefore, breathing plays a very important role in our transformation since we want to charge our bodies with a higher concentration of biophotons in order to become more alive and happy.

Because our consciousness is directly related to the concentration of biophotons, we can also train ourselves to direct the inhaled biophoton-energy by will power to a certain body region. This can acutally cause bioplasma to move to the desired location of our body.

Therefore, this consciously guided breath with the enclosed biophoton-energy is extremely important and useful for all transformation exercises.

Equally relevant is the conscious exhalation. While exhaling, we can imagine  sending away with the breathing stream all uncomfortable feelings and negative thoughts. This is ultimately nothing  but practically applied quantum physics because feelings and thoughts represent specific electromagnetic fields i.e. photons. This breathing method is very old and has been practiced by the Indian Yogis and Egyptian priests for millennia.

*To the exercise performance*

For the breathing exercises that we come to know now, it is good if we are not interrupted and do not have any disturbing noises intrude on us from the outside. It is equally important that we close our eyes during this time because if we are in the everyday state of our consciousness, we allow ourselves time and again to be distracted by the sight of our surroundings.

But during these exercises we want to learn to give all our attention to what is happening within ourselves. We want to get to know ourselves better: our body, our feelings and our thoughts and behind all of that of course we want to discover our happy original state.

Basically, we should  either  breath in  and out through

the nose or in through the nose and out through the mouth. The nose with her sinuses is not only here for smelling but firstly, the incoming air is already heated here and secondly, a part of the bioplasma contained in the air is already being absorbed by our body through the mucous membranes of the nasal cavities.

When we have a cold, we can and must make an exception to this rule of course. If our nose is blocked by a cold, we should be careful not to breathe in air that is too icy through the mouth since otherwise a cold could spread to the lungs.

And here another important note: If we do our exercises indoors, we must provide the room with fresh air prior to the exercises. We always air the space well ahead of our exercises.

# EXERCISES FOR CONSCIOUS BREATHING

*Harmonious inhaling and exhaling*

**The starting position:** We are seated as upright as possible on a chair which is not too soft. We draw our shoulders backwards very slightly – without much tension, so that our head does not rest in front of our chest like a crane jib, but instead rests above it. If we were to drop a vertical line straight down from our chin, where it hits our chest is the area of the thymus gland. This is exactly the place between the nipples in men and the hollow between the two breasts in women. The upper arms hang down vertically by the sides of the body and the forearms and hands rest horizontally on our thighs.

Initially, this position is more pleasant if we lean on and cling to a chair back with our straight spine. Later we can assume this position relaxed on a stool without a backrest – but this is not so important at the moment. We relax our chest and abdomen.

**The breathing intervall:** We close (if possible) the eyes. Then we start to inhale slowly and deeply and to exhale. For this there is a little trick: First of all exhale fully and then start with the inhaling. For each sequence, we allow ourselves about 10 seconds, with a total of 20 seconds. In the beginning, we focus on the inhaling and exhaling and try to let the air flow in and out just as fast as it takes to meet the time of about 20 seconds for each breath cycle. If we are to fast on inhaling or exhaling, we cannot keep the time interval. Very quietly and harmoniously, we breath in and out, completely symmetrical.

**The diaphragmatic breathing:** When we have found a harmonious rhythm of breathing, we observe where in the body we are breathing. Are we only lifting and dropping the chest while inhaling or is the abdomen moving forward and coming back as well while exhaling, just as it happens with diaphragmatic breathing? Many people who have repressed unpleasant feelings in their belly are chest- or so called flat-breathers for whom it is certainly difficult to extend the respiratory rhythm to 20 seconds. If we become aware of our breathing pattern, we now want to practice breathing into our abdomen consciously. We should get into the habit of this diaphragmatic breathing, because it supplies us much more efficiently with oxygen and bioplasma than the flat respiration. Also, our lungs can expand downwards more effectively and thus can exchange more air per breath. So we become more alive.

**Extending the cycle:** After having set our focus on diaphragmatic breathing, we try to extend a respiratory cycle to 30 seconds in total. This is achieved not only by breathing down into the diaphragm and thereby bulging our belly but also by extending our chest deliberately (completely consciously) each time we inhale until we reach the full volume.

This exercise should be performed for about ten minutes – or perhaps, even a few minutes longer. We should repeat it a few days in a row to get into the habit of making use of our entire lung volume.

Also in everyday life, we should watch our breath every now and then consciously. If anything excites us, it is very helpful to breath deeply and calmly. This creates a conscious connection with the world outside as a whole and can be done wonderfully in nature, in the garden or wherever we feel comfortable.

*Guiding the breath energy*

**The starting position:** We assume the same starting point as described at the beginning of the previous exercise. Then we bring our breath cycle back to about 30 seconds and breath deeply and quietly in and out.

**Guiding the breath:** In this exercise we want to learn to pay attention not only to our breath but also to observe our thoughts and feelings. If we perceive an unpleasant feeling, we try to locate it in our body. Maybe it is a discomfort in the stomach, in the abdomen, in the chest or wherever. We then imagine that we absorb happy energy into us while inhaling and direct it to the point where we feel uncomfortable. On the exhale, we imagine that the discomfort leaves our body. With the next inhalation we get another new dose of happiness and so on, and so on. Maybe some anger or a negative thought bothers us. This happens naturally in the head and we can imagine that the inhaled happy energy flows into our head, washes around the bad thoughts and these leave while exhaling. Let us just invite happiness to come into us.

This exercise as well, can be done for ten minutes or as long as we would like.

# RELAX AND LET GO

Due to the stress of everyday life, whether at work, at school, in the family or in relationships, many people have become accustomed to repressing negative experiences, where they suffered psychological injuries and the associated feelings. This results in tension in the muscles and connective tissues. Poor posture while sitting or standing can lead through imbalances to chronic tension in all areas of the body as well. All of the above cause blockages in the energy flow of the bioplasma and reduces our wellbeing, our vitality and our quality of life.

Often people are not aware of how tense they are. If we touch our neck and shoulder muscles for example, many of us will probably notice a strong tenseness or chronic strain. Very often even a small amount of pressure onto a muscle is enough to elicit pain. As a result of the permanent strain, the muscle tissue becomes too acidic. The associated electron deficiency prevents a high bioplasma concentration from being created there and the acidic chemical environment leads to additional problems in the form of deposits. This takes a lot of life energy from our bodies.

Since we want to free ourselves of such loads by transformation, it is very important to learn how to relax. Anyone who has ever taken a purring domestic cat in his arms, is surprised at how relaxed such an animal is, when it feels comfortable. If one raises a paw, it falls down like a rock when released.

Relaxing always has something to do with letting go. We not only release a strained muscle, but we also want to let go of the dull feelings connected to tension and this works even better, if we exhale consciously and deeply while relaxing. Like this we allow the disharmonious energy patterns to leave our body during exhalation. So we combine the following exercises to relax and let go with the breathing exercises that we have learned in the previous section.

*Tensing up – relax – let go*

**The starting position:** We stand upright, feet approximately half a metre apart, our legs stretched.

**Hooking:** If we want to learn to relax, it is adviseable first of all to tense up with awareness – every muscle in the face, in the throat and neck, in the shoulders, in the upper and lower ams and hands, in the abdominal part, in the buttocks, in the thighs, knees, calves and feet. We take a deep breath, hold the air in, then tighten all parts of the body mentioned above – with all your energy. In this way we are standing there, ready for extremes, no matter who is coming – nothing is going to knock us over.

**Relax:** After 15 seconds we start to slowly exhale while relaxing all the muscles that we have previously tightened up. On the exhale we let all aggression escape. We become completely soft and peaceful.

We can repeat this process a few times. After that it is best to continue the exercise lying down.

**Lying down:** For this, we lie flat on the floor – not on a mattress, a bed or a couch. We can spread a blanket on the ground and support our head with a thin cushion,  so that we can lie loose. The legs are stretched out straight and the feet angled slightly outward as far as they are pulled by gravity. Our arms are outstretched along our body with the palms downwards without tension. If it is too chilly for us, we cover ourselves with a thin but warm blanket.

**Tensening up and relaxing:** First we close our  eyes. Now we repeat the exercise which we did earlier while standing. So, first take a deep breath, hold the air for about 15 seconds while  tightening up all the muscles. Then exhale slowly and allow the muscles to relax.

**Perceiving and release:** After repeating this exercise a few times while lying down, we then go one step further and identify what feelings we perceive in ourselves. If these are uncomfortable things, such as anger at someone, rage or hurt, then these emotions become quite clear during the tension phase. We let go of them while exhaling and relaxing.

If we have pleasant experiences, we invite such pleasurable sensations with futher inhalation and do not tense ourselves up any more. With the slow and deep exhaling we let go of any other tension in our body.

After we have done such an exercise for ten minutes, we feel noticeably better. Our thoughts are clearer, we feel fresher and more balanced.

We want to accept ourselves as we are. We are pleased to be able to do these exercises and for having the opportunity to develop ourselves. We are grateful.

# DEEP RELAXATION

The exercise of deep relaxation described below, is an important preparation for some spiritual transformation- and meditation methods, which we will learn in the third chapter in order to get a deep access to our subconsciousness and our soul with the hidden information stored there.

This exercise leads us into a deep state of relaxation. I have often noticed in my workshops that some participants fall asleep during this. For people who have problems with falling asleep, this method is a particularly effective antidote.

*Relaxing autosuggestion*

**The starting position:** The execution of the deep relaxation is only worthwhile when lying down.

Since it is often followed by a longer quiet transformation or meditation method, it is useful in any case to cover oneself with a thin but warm blanket, so that one does not get cold during the session.

People who use this method to deal with their sleeping problems can of course curl up in their bed.

In any case, we take the same position lying down as in the previous floor exercise.

**Consciously breathing:** First of all we concentrate on our breathing. We breath deeply and calmly in and out like we have learnt in the first breathing section (p. 26 ff.).

**Use the imagination:** Now, we imagine that every body part on which we focus our attention, becomes very heavy. The text for the deep relaxation can be played either from an audio CD, or we can have a partner read it to us who will guide us in deep relaxation, or we can read it to ourselves or think of it in our heads. For each body part that we want to relax thouroughly, we give ourselves about five to ten seconds time. We imagine that exactly what we are hearing or thinking is what is happening.

Text of the deep relaxation (I-form):

> My right foot relaxes and becomes completely heavy.
> My right lower leg with my shin and calf relaxes
  and becomes completely heavy.
> My right knee relaxes and becomes completely heavy.
> My right thigh relaxes and becomes completely heavy.
> My left foot relaxes and becomes completely heavy.
> My left lower leg with my shin and calf relaxes
  and becomes completely heavy.

> My left knee relaxes and becomes completely heavy.

> My left thigh relaxes and becomes completely heavy.

> My pelvis relaxes and becomes completely heavy.
> My tailbone relaxes and becomes completely heavy.
> My belly relaxes and becomes completely heavy.
> My lumbar vertebrae relax and become completely heavy.

> My solar plexus relaxes and becomes completely heavy.

> My back relaxes and becomes completely heavy.
> My chest relaxes and becomes completely heavy.
> My shoulders relax and become completely heavy.

> My right upper arm relaxes and becomes completely heavy.

> My right forearm relaxes and becomes completely heavy.

> My right hand relaxes and becomes completely heavy.

> My left upper arm relaxes and becomes completely heavy.

> My left forearm relaxes and becomes completely heavy.

> My left hand relaxes and becomes completely heavy.

> My neck relaxes and becomes completely heavy.

> My cervical vertebrae relax and become completely heavy.

> My throat relaxes and becomes completely heavy.

> My chin relaxes and becomes completely heavy.

> My mouth relaxes and becomes completely heavy.

> My nose relaxes and becomes completely heavy.

> My eyes relax and become completely heavy.

> My cheeks relax and become completely heavy.

> My forehead relaxes and becomes completely heavy.

> My head relaxes and becomes completely heavy.

**Text of the deep relaxation (you-form):**

> Your right foot relaxes and becomes completely heavy.

> Your right lower leg with shin and calf relaxes and becomes completely heavy.

> Your right knee relaxes and becomes completely heavy.

> Your right thigh relaxes and becomes completely heavy.

> Your left foot relaxes and becomes completely heavy.

> Your left lower leg with shin and calf relaxes and becomes completely heavy.

> Your left knee relaxes and becomes completely heavy.

> Your left thigh relaxes and becomes completely heavy.

> Your pelvis relaxes and becomes completely heavy.

> Your tailbone relaxes and becomes completely heavy.

> Your belly relaxes and becomes completely heavy.

> Your lumbar vertebrae relax and become completely heavy.

> Your solar plexus relaxes and becomes completely heavy.

> Your back relaxes and becomes completely heavy.
> Your chest relaxes and becomes completely heavy.
> Your shoulders relax and become completely heavy.

> Your right upper arm relaxes and becomes completely heavy.

> Your right forearm relaxes and becomes completely heavy.

> Your right hand relaxes and becomes completely heavy.

> Your left upper arm relaxes and becomes completely heavy.

> Your left forearm relaxes and becomes completely heavy.

> Your left hand relaxes and becomes completely heavy.

> Your neck relaxes and becomes completely heavy.
> Your cervical vertebrae relax and become completely heavy.

> Your throat relaxes and becomes completely heavy.
> Your chin relaxes and becomes completely heavy.
> Your mouth relaxes and becomes completely heavy.
> Your nose relaxes and becomes completely heavy.
> Your eyes relax and become completely heavy.
> You cheeks relax and become completely heavy.
> Your forehead relaxes and becomes completely heavy.
> Your head relaxes and becomes completely heavy.

If we are still awake after this deep relaxation and direct our whole attention inwards and only observe our body´s reactions, feelings and thoughts, we are ready for a deep insight into our soul. We deal with this further leading meditation in chapter three.

## INTENSE NOSE BREATHING

A particularly effective method to very quickly and strongly recharge the body with bioplasma is the intense nose breathing. It is advisable to use this method with caution, not to overdo it and make sure you are not alone the first times, but apply it with a partner or in a group.

**The starting position:** Before we start, we prepare ourselves a place on the ground, place a small pillow there for our head, spread a blanket on which we can lay on later and keep another blanket ready, with which we can then cover ourselfs with.

Furthermore, it is a good thing to put a glass of water next to us, because what follows is a small „sporting" event.

**Intense nose breathing:** We stand upright and whilst being relaxed begin to inhale very intensely and exhale through our nose as fast as we can with our mouth shut. We always need to keep the mouth closed. In the rythm of the fast breathing cycle we rock and bounce with our knees and move our hands up and down with ease. With some practice we get into a harmonious rythmic movement, which supports the rapid breathing cycle.

On the first time we can try to endure this intense nose breathing for about five minutes. For later practisings of this method, we can improve to approximately ten to fifteen minutes.


**On the ground, self-perception:** At the end we make ourselves comfortable on the ground and assume the prone position, which was described in the first floor exercise (p. 32 ff). Now, we breath calmly and deeply in and out. We close our eyes and observe what is going on inside of us. Our body is at this point enriched not only with oxygen but also with lots of biophotons. We now have the opportunity to precisely observe the points where our body's energy flow is blocked off. Due to the higher concentration of biophotons our inner perception is increased.


**Effects and possible side effects:** It may happen that we experience, aside from reactions in the body, intense feelings as well. Perhaps, some tears may come. When it is all good, we can allow all of this to come up by just continuously inhaling and exhaling calmly, relaxing and letting go as we have been practicing earlier.

With each time of practice, we will be able to keep up the intense nose breathing longer. It can also happen that we feel a tingling or prickling sensation during or after an intense nose breathing, usually in the hands and forearms, as if we were to go numb there. Do not worry, these unfamiliar reactions do not continue for long. They come about because the energy pathways in the body are not yet used to transporting such amounts of bioplasma. Our energy system is now beginning to grow and to open up and for that reason we will burst through it again and again.

In some people the hands clench, the palms pull together like paws and it is also possible that dizziness occurs. In case of such (hyperventilation-) symptoms one should immediately go on with a calm rhythm of breathing. A rapid solution to the unpleasant cramps is provided if one inhales and exhales calmly in a paper bag.

Some feel fresh and like they are reborn in the aftermath of this exercise. With it we have experienced that there are still boundaries in our energy system, but it also means, that we have development possibilities and that of course we want to realise this potential.

# 2. BODY EXERCISES

## AN INNER BODY CLEANSING

Our body is the Quantum Temple. Therefore, any transformation process cannot be initiated without body oriented methods. Unconsciously, we have many suppressed feelings and emotional pain stored away in our bodies. In order to rid ourselves in terms of energy of these burdens and to achieve a higher biophoton concentration and with that a higher state of consciousness, we need physical exercises and appropriate methods with which to bring out the supressed experiences from our body. It may at first not be pleasant to have to look at repressed uncomfortable experiences again, but there is no way around it.

Somebody with all their repressed feelings is like the home of a „hoarder" before the transformation, which has not been tidied up and cleaned in years and is full of all kinds of trash and useless objects.

In order to breathe freely again and make it so our body becomes a vessel for light and happiness, we have to make room and remove all debris.

# SHAKING AND LOOSENING UP

The following is a highly effective method which is suitable to dissolve blockages in the lower four energy centers of the body, in the stomach and chest area. Experience has shown that this is the place where the most energy blockages caused by repressed emotions such as anger, resignation, sadness and fear can be found. This method can accompany and support the development and purification of the energy system over a longer period of time as often as once a day. „Shaking" is a belly-dance-like movement, in which particularly the pelvic region is agitated. Hereby, the body moves in its vertical axis back and forth with rapid movements. In doing so, it is crucial to let everything be loose - especially the belly area.

**Remove blockades:** Most people get sharp pain quite promptly by doing this exercise for the first time, mainly in the abdominal area, in the midriff, the diaphragm and on the sides of the chest. They then say: „I get stitches in the side." However, these side stitches are nothing but the blockades in the energy system, which are now felt through the strong movement and want to dissolve themselves. While shaking, it is important to accept the pain that occurs up to a tolerable level and to see through the mechanism and let go of whatever leads to cramping. Nobody should overextend this. Through the individual adjustment of the intensity of shaking, you can approach exactly the point, where the pain remains well observable. It is now crucial to focus all the attention on to the painful area and try to breathe into this place. Thus, the tension can be resolved at this point.

The pain is caused by an accumulation of electromagnetic energy (biophotons) that is exchanged between the body's electrons. As soon as the energy channels are free again, the pain is resolved, and the light energy can flow freely from electron to electron.

It has been confirmed in hundreds of experiments with my measuring method for detecting the bioplasma (see chapter 6) that the energy pathways are so to speak cleared by the application of body- and spirit-based transformation methods.

Most people will hold on very strongly, when they first start with the shaking, until they realise slowly how to dissolve the tension. Many make the observation over a period of time that an energy blockade, which was first felt in the stomach, wanders consistently further up. This comes from bioplasma now flowing from the upper energy centers into the abdominal area to replenish the locally exposed energy holes and blockades. Thus, the upper energy centers run empty for a short time, because the selfhealing powers of the human energy system are of course limited at the beginning.

**Shaking free:** In order to shake free the heart center, the chest should be expanded by raising the hands.

For this purpose the upper arms are extended laterally away outwards from the torso and the forearms with the hands stretched upwards approximately at a right angle. The upper body is then twisted during shaking in the opposite direction to the pelvis. This method is a lot of fun with lively, rhythmic music.

Relaxing and perceiving: After shaking, which is practiced for maybe five to ten minutes, it is good to lie down and relax. If we then have areas and points in our body that feel empty of energy, it is helpful to put our hands there and breathe deeply and calmly. Now we should direct all our attention inwards and observe our thoughts and feelings.

After an intense shaking phase it is possible that violent emotional relapses flood through our body and we may break out in tears or also notice old, repressed anger rises within us. Simply allow, ever more relaxing and continued breathing and meet all the feelings and thoughts that wash through your system with love . The most important thing is that we love and forgive ourselves for everything, if there is something to be forgiven.

Everybody who practices this exercise for a while, will notice that more and more tension is dissolving and a higher vitality level is reached each time the exercise is done. We are much more alive and no longer waste a large part of our life energy to keep uncomfortable emotions in check and out of our consciousness.

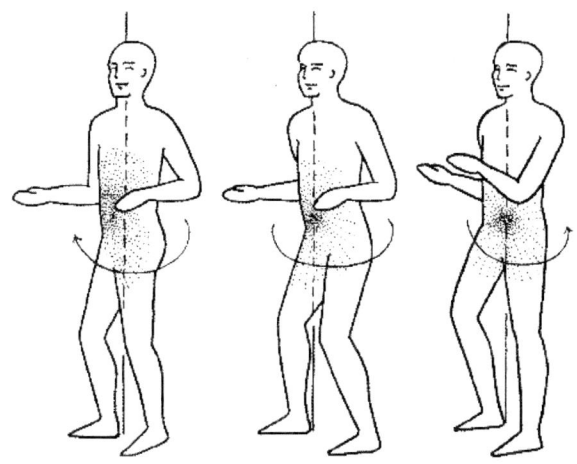

a) Shaking of the pelvic and abdominal area

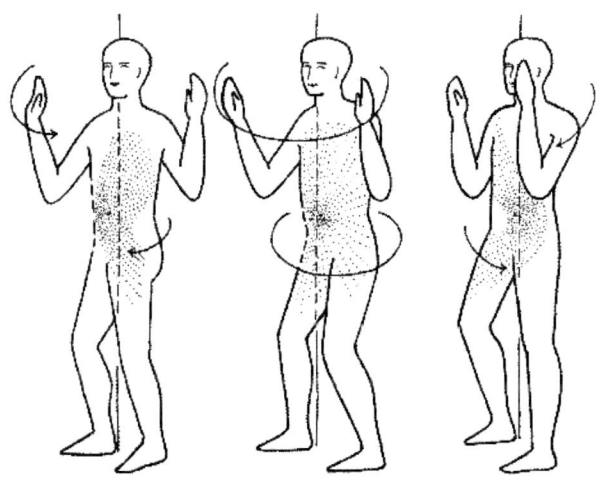

b) Shaking of the upper body with simultaneous movement
   of the belly area in the opposite direction

45

# STRETCHING EXERCISES

From the Traditional Chinese Medicine (TCM) it is known that our body is crisscrossed by energy pathways, called acupuncture meridians. At certain locations of the body, the acupuncture points, the energetic status can also be measured electrically. If a meridian can carry a lot of biophoton energy, we measure a higher electrical conductivity at the corresponding acupuncture points. In this case, there are more free electrons and thus also more biophotons.

The stretching exercises described below, which I have developped from various traditions, are very effective to enhance the flow of energy in our bodies. Through these exercises, the energy channels are cleaned free so to speak.

Some meridians are also related to the metabolism of our body and therefore the detoxification functions of our system are stimulated by some of these exercises. With regular use, an increased detoxification and cleansing of the body are noticeable.

**To the exercise performance:** It is important not to try to achieve a stronger stretching effect of certain body parts through rocking or similar movements while performing these exercises but to do them in a way so that the strains are clearly felt. Often though, we will only become aware of how tense we really are in some places by doing them.

When we have taken a stretching position, it is very helpful to breath deeply during it and to draw our breath (in spirit) to the places where we perceive a tension or a spasm. Since the air molecules that we inhale, are also enriched with photon energy – in the form of excited molecular states – we supply our body parts with photon energy through every breath and help them to increase the biophoton concentration.

It is recommended to always start with the exercise number one for the Central and Governing Vessel and then follow with the other exercises one after the other in the given order. Everyone can choose the best suited individual version of the two or three variants given per exercise. Each one of them should be performed for about a minute.

*1. Central and Governing Vessel*

(Equalization and distribution function in the meridian system)

a) **Floor:** Sitting in the vault, bend the upper body straight ahead out from the pelvis and shift the weight forward with the help of the arms. At the same time stretch the feet for enforcement and tighten and circle them.

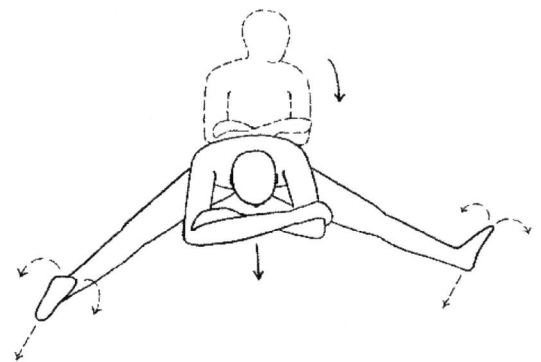

**As a partner exercise:** Sitting in front of each other on the floor, the soles of both partners touching. Grasp each others hands and gyrate easily with the upper bodies.

b) **Chair:** Sitting in the straddle position, bend the upper body forward and then do as in a).

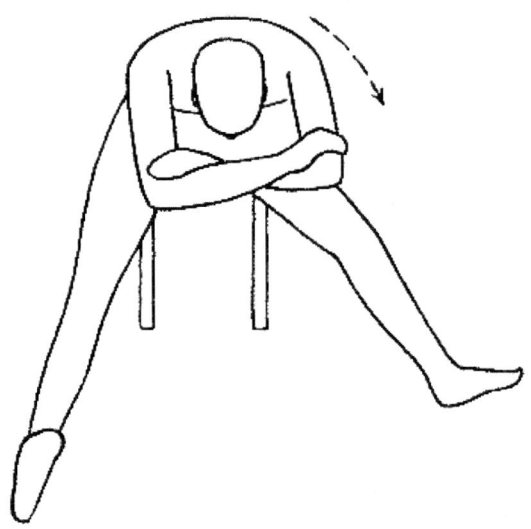

b) ((Grafik 4b scribble, 448.jpg))

## 2. Spleen and Stomach Meridian

(Digestive function)

a) **Floor 1:** In the heel seat – holding the thighs parallel – bend the upper body backwards to the ground. The elongation occurs in the region of the abdomen and the thighs. Extend the arms backwards over the head to achieve an enhanced stretching. Allow deep in- and exhaling. With each exhale let the stretching go further.

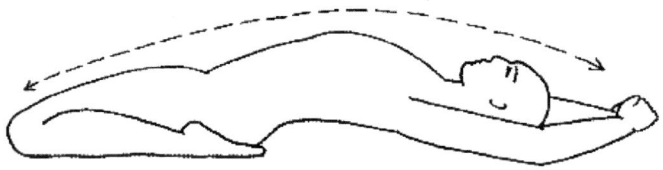

b) **Floor 2:** After a) perform the counter movement for relaxation: In the heel seat bend your upper body forward until the forehead touches the ground. The arms are parallel to the legs.

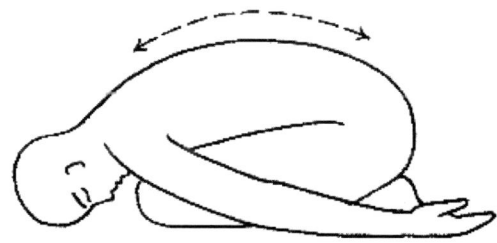

c) **Variant to exercise a) and b):** While lying down, bend one leg and place it across over the other leg, so that the angled knee touches the ground. During this, the shoulders should stay in

49

contact with the ground. Meet the knee with the hand to help it. Then turn around and repeat the whole thing with the other leg.

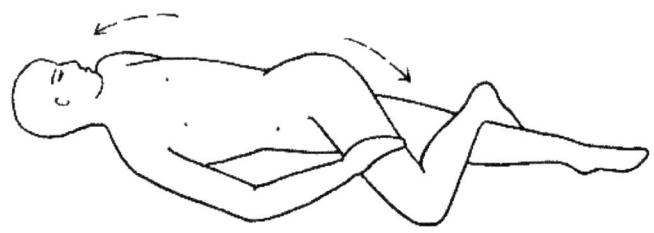

**d) Chair:** With legs crossed over and shifting the upper body, including the arms, to one side, in the opposite direction of the legs, move backwards.

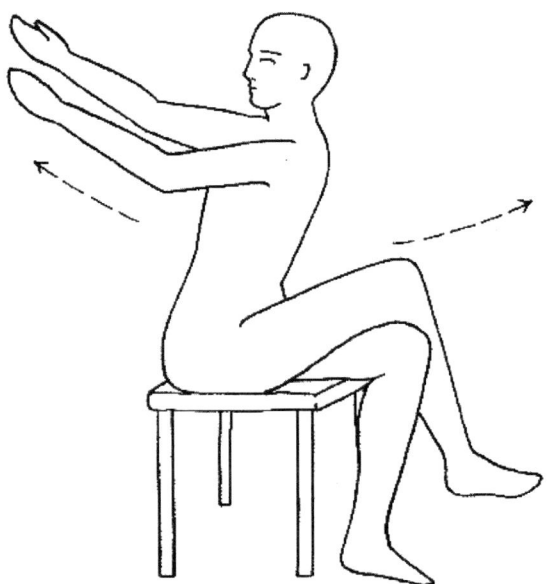

## 3. Heart Meridian

(Stretching of the chest, stimulation of the circulation)

a)    **Standing:** With a stretched neck pose (head extended upwards) lift both arms simultaneously to the rear. During this, bend the hands outwards, so that an expansion from the sternum to the fingertips takes place. In- and exhale deeply while doing so. When inhaling gradually lift the arms up slowly, remaining stretched out, until the fingertips meet over your head. Finally bring the hands to the heart level (in front of your chest) and draw your attention to the inside.

b) **Chair:** In case of circulatory problems, perform the stretching while sitting down as described in a).

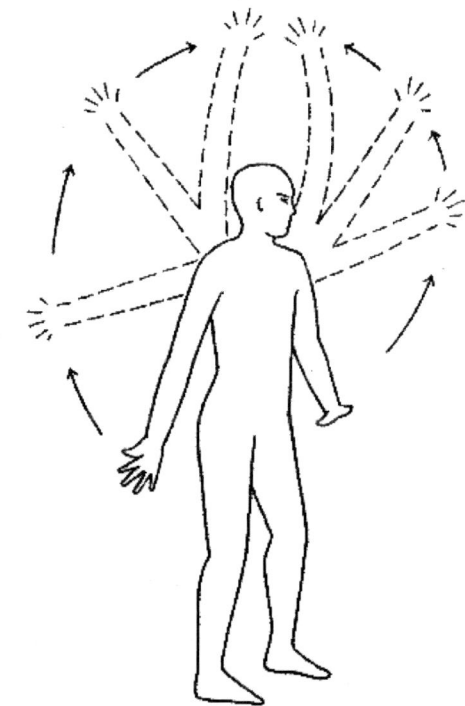

*4. Heart - Small Intestine - Meridian*

(Control of the metabolism)

**Floor:** While sitting down, put the soles of your feet together and hold them with both hands. On the exhale bend forward from the pelvic area, the nose pointing in the direction of your feet. The elongation is noticeable on the insides of the thighs. Hold the position and allow more stretching through deep breathing.

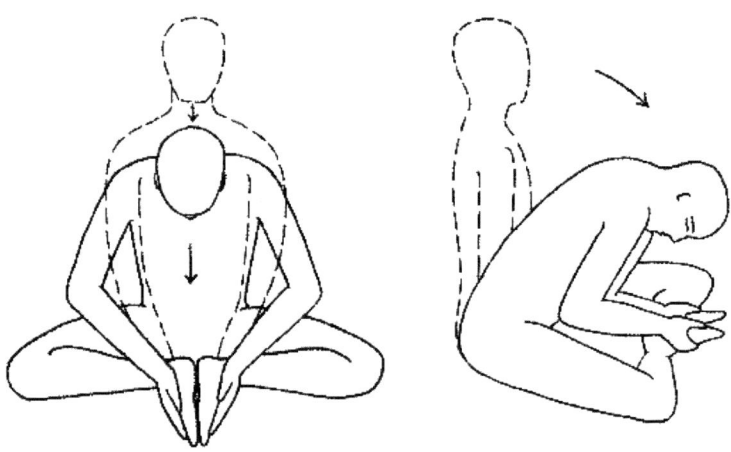

*5. Kidney – Bladder – Meridian*

(Excretory organs and cleaning function)

a ) **Floor:** From the upright sitting posture stretch the legs out parallel without effort. Exhale and bend forward with the head in direction of the knees. The stretching is felt along the bottom of the legs. For amplification of the stretching, reach to the calves, ankles or to the soles of your feet with your hands. Breath deeply, relax into this position.

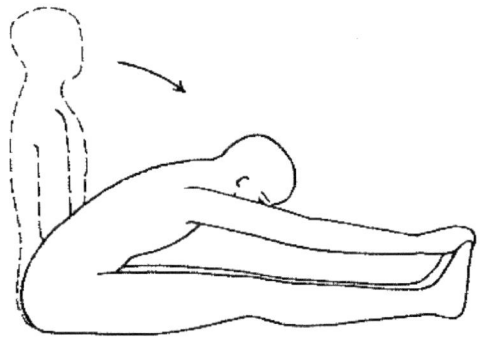

b) **Standing:** Search hold on a window sill or on a dresser with outstretched arms and straight legs. The upper body bends forward towards the window sill.

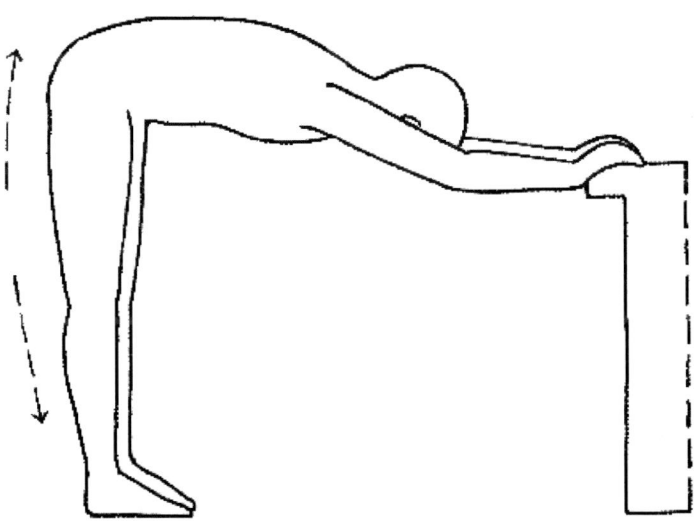

## 6. Triple Heater

(Circulation)

**Standing:** The hands hooked with the fingers behind the back – one hand coming from above, the other one from below, so that the stretching is felt in the arms. Inhale and exhale deeply. Then repeat the exercise crossed over. This time one hand comes from above, the other hand from below.

**For the exercise performance:** If it is not possible to hook the hands with the fingers, guide them carefully and as close together as possible. One can also take a sock or a scarf to help out. Hold the ends of the stocking with boths hands and merge them as close as possible behind yor back.

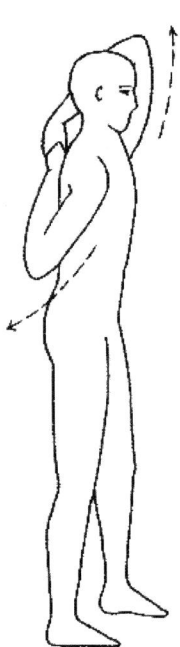

*7. Gallbladder Meridian*

(In the thigh area)

Floor: When seated, one leg is bent flat on the ground, facing inward. The other leg crosses over the first one, so that the knees are above each other as much as possible. Bend forward with the upper body from the pelvic area until the stretching is felt in the buttocks and the thighs. Then change position – switch legs.

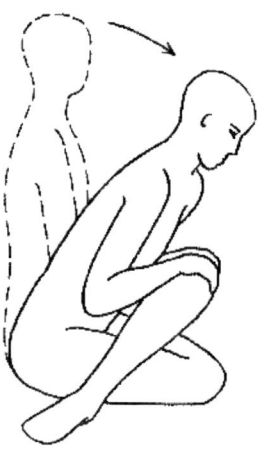

*8. Liver and Gallbladder Meridian*

(Storage and transfer function, detoxification)

a ) **Floor:** From the seated straddle position bend one leg backwards inside. Grip the other extended leg from the inside underneath the calf with your hand and with the other hand slowly describe a semicircle over your head until the upper body is bent sideways towards the stetched out leg. Breath deeply into the lateral expansion of the upper body. Then repeat the exercise the other way around, so this time bend the other leg and with the other arm describe the semi-arc over your head, etc.

b) **Chair:** When seated, bend one arm over your head, so that the side of the arched arm is stretched. Move the other, free arm in front of your chest and abdominal area in the opposite direction in order to balance. Execute this exercise also symmetrically to the other side.

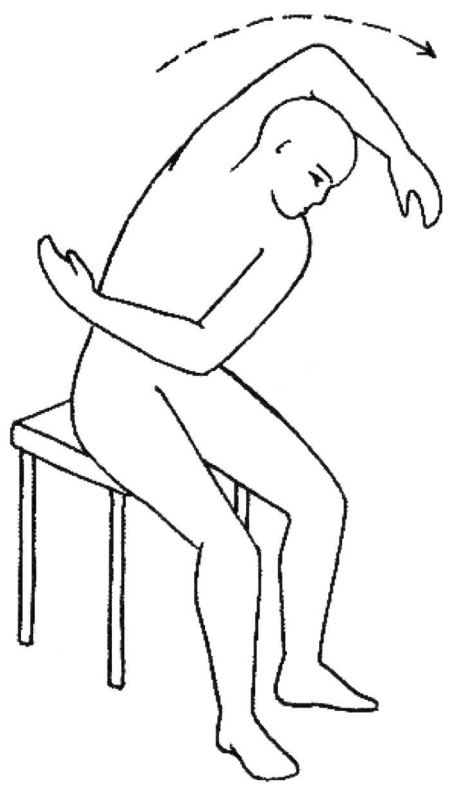

## 9. Lung and Large Intestine Meridian

(Intake of energy through respiration / excretion)

a ) **Standing:** One hand is holding the thumb of the other hand behind the back. Inhale deeply, exhale slowly, thereby bending forwards from the waist and extending the arms, in which the stretching ist noticed, upwards and forwards as far as possible. Hold the position and breathe. Repeat the same thing with the other arm and hand.

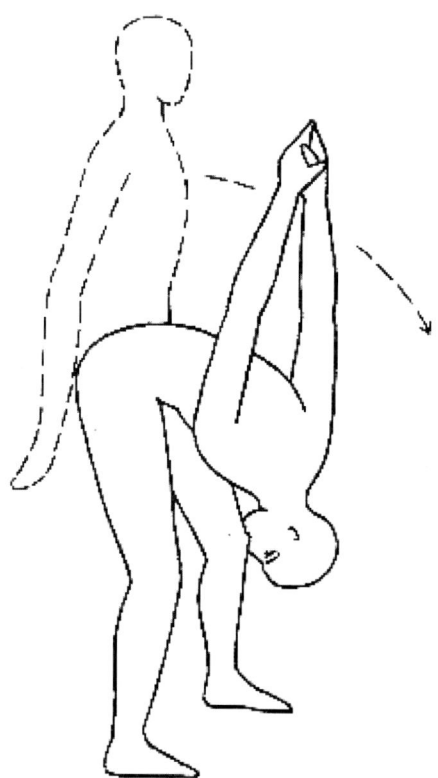

**b)**    **Chair:** Perform like a) in a sitting position. The exercise can take place instead of on a chair or standing up squatting in the heal seat.

## 10. Final exercise

**a) Floor:** Go into the neck balance until the main weight rests on your shoulders and the neck. Shortly stay in this position which causes a strain on the neck. Then stretch the legs over your head until your feet touch the ground. Grasp the soles of your feet with your hands and bring the knees as close as possible to the body. Persist in this ball position, breath and relax into it. The entire spine is extended. After this straighten your legs upwards.

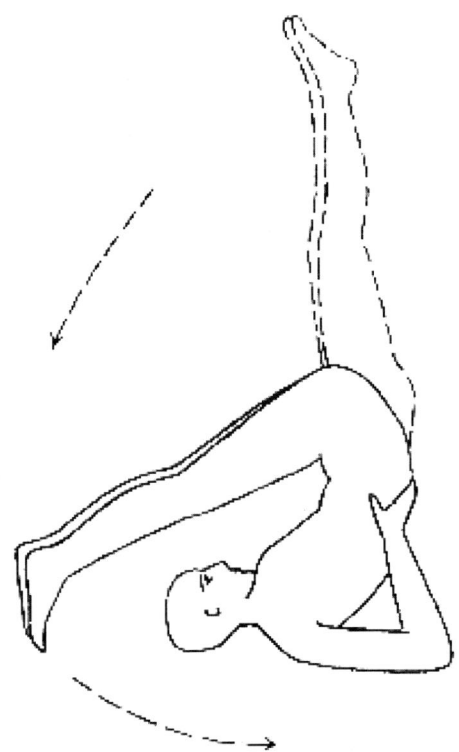

Meanwhile your hands are stretched to touch your feet. Gently slide down, vertebra by vertebra. Through the contact of the hands with the feet you set and vary the pace of the unrolling yourself.

b) **Chair:** Intertwine both hands behind your head. First bend your head and let it sink towards the ground through the weight of your hands, then slowly bend the entire torso and back forward – just by the weight of your hands and arms as well.

Remain in this position for a while. Feel your spine and imagine the whole spinal cord from the tailbone to the cervical vertebrae in your mind. At the end slowly rise one vertebra after the other.

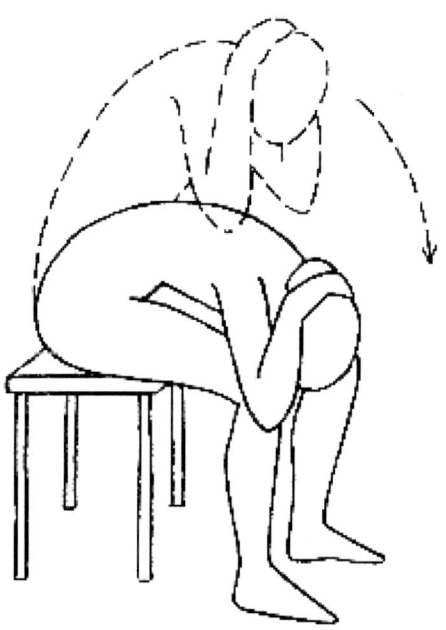

# MASSAGES

One could easily devote an entire book on the theme of massage, but we want to limit ourselves here to a few massage techniques that anyone can practice by themselves.

The body oriented methods that we have already seen in previous sections, are quite suitable to solve many of the tensions in ourseves, especially if we reflect on their emotional background and have learned to loosen up and let go.

However, some muscle tensions and hardenings are so great that they can be helped further by targeted massaging of the affected parts and muscles of the body. All the more effective we can then dissolve the loosened tension with the breathing and stretching exercises. The massage is therefore complimentary to the methods described above.

**Massage oils:** An important and downright indispensable tool for the massage is the massage oil. In health food stores such oils are usually offered, partly refined with effective essential oils. Here, everyone can choose a massage oil with an appealing fragrance.
So, before we begin a massage treatment, we should rub the massage oil on both our hands as well as on the areas of the body to be massaged.

**With partner:** Massages are performed optimally in a partner exercise for two. While in principle it is possible to massage ourselves on the reflex zones of the hands and feet, a massage shows a stronger relaxing effect if the person treated can concentrate on the breathing, feeling inwards, relaxing and letting go.

During the massage, especially if a painful, tense spot is treated, it is useful to remember the breathing exercises, where we have focused our breath on a certain area in our body. The method of breath guiding can be used to better provide a massaged part with bioplasma. In this way, we support the transformation process that has been initiated through the massage.

About the performing of a massage: A massage of the entire back region, including shoulders and neck muscles is usually particularly beneficial. These are often very tense in many people, mostly due to poor posture. In a back massage especially the muscle parts to the right and left of the spine should be treated.

While massaging, the masseur should excert a firm pressure with his thumbs and fingers on the spot to be treated in a circular motion in order to loosen up the tense muscle tissue. After such an intense loosening up massage, it is important and also very soothing to the massaged person, if the treated parts are gently stroked with the palms. Like this, the bioplasma can be distributed harmoniously across the whole area.

It is a common misconception that a massage is especially good if it is also very painful. This is wrong, because our consciousness and our perception withdraw immediately from an area if a pain becomes unbearable.

It is better if masseur and massaged person communicate clearly during the massage, concerning the applied massage pressure, to ensure it is not too week or not too strong. Ideally, a tolerable pain is produced by the massage, into which the person massaged can consciously breathe and relax. The point is not to separate the massaged body part from the total sensation but to integrate it consciously into the own sensory awareness. Like this, we can obtain a higher well-being if we face the old painful experiences, but not by achieving new records in bearing particularly severe pain. We do not want to torment our bodies, but set them free from blockades, so that the happy energy can flood anywhere within us.

**Detoxification:** The massage allows for better blood flow within the treated region and thus contributes to a better supply of oxygen and all other substances that the blood transports. Waste products and other toxins deposited in cramped tissue are mobilized and eliminated more rapidly.

It is recommended that a person drinks a sufficient amount of liquids – preferably clear water – before and after a massage. Like this, the detoxification process, which is fueled by the massage, gets additional support. Cramped muscle tissue is often too acidic and reacts more sensitive than relaxed tissue. Here the pain threshold is very low.

Through a massage, violent and pent-up emotions, which were tucked away in the tension of muscles can be released.Therefore, one should allow oneself enough time after the treatment to observe all the sensations in ones interior and harmonize them by the learned breathing techniques.

Reflexology massage: in addition to the massage of various body parts such as back, neck, shoulders, abdomen and chest area, the massage of the hand and foot reflexology points offers itself to us, as depicted on the following two pages. Through the massage of the shown reflex zones, we can affect certain organs of the body in terms of their enery. By the light pressure and circular motion of the thumb the reflex zones can be activated. The stimulating effect on the corresponding organs is often amazing.

Thus, I have experienced in my workshops again and again that people who have had digestive problems or suffered from a chronic constipation, were showing through the massage of the reflex zones of the metabolic organs, especially the ones of the small and large intestines, very spontaneous reactions in the affected organs, and therefore sought out quite quickly a certain place to relieve themselves. When massaging the reflex zones of the large intestine one should make sure to massage with one's thumb along the transport direction of the colon. So, be sure to observe the massage direction.

This is particularly true for a belly massage as well. For on most people (anatomical exceptions excluded) we should massage up on the right side of the abdomen to about the level of the lower rib cage (Colon ascendens), then along between the navel and the sternum from right to left (Colon transversalis) and finally down on the left side of the rib cage into the left area below the navel (Colon descendens). Like this we can optimise the

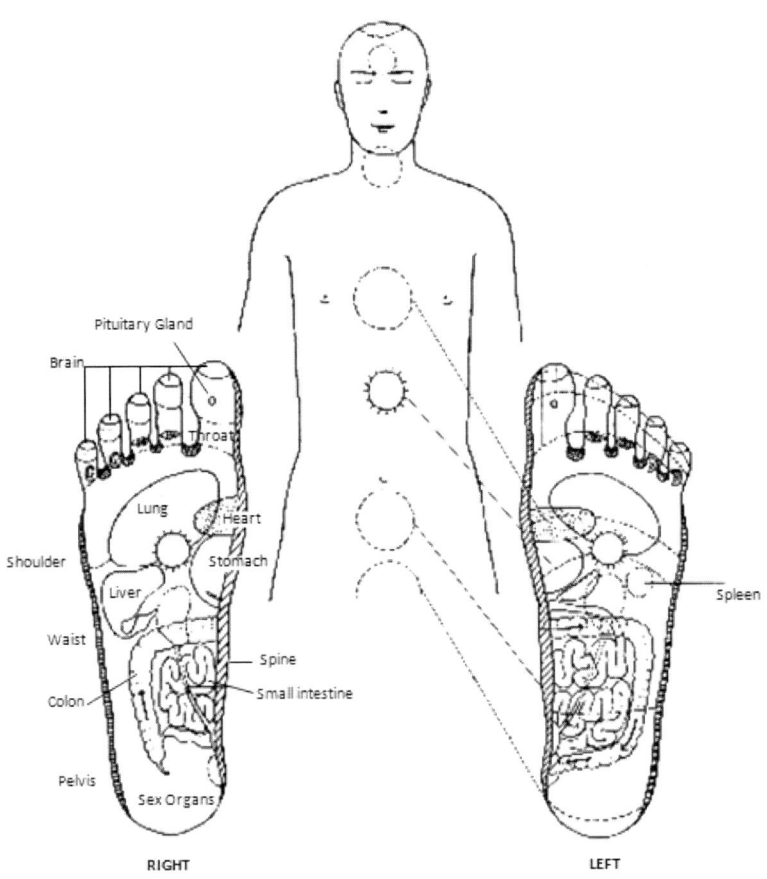

digestive functions through an abdominal massage. Massages are therefore an important tool for our spiritual transformation, because they can help us to transport back to the surface of our consciousness, old painful experiences that we have repressed in certain areas of our body in order to process and transform them now in a loving and healing atmosphere and with a conciliatory inner attitude.

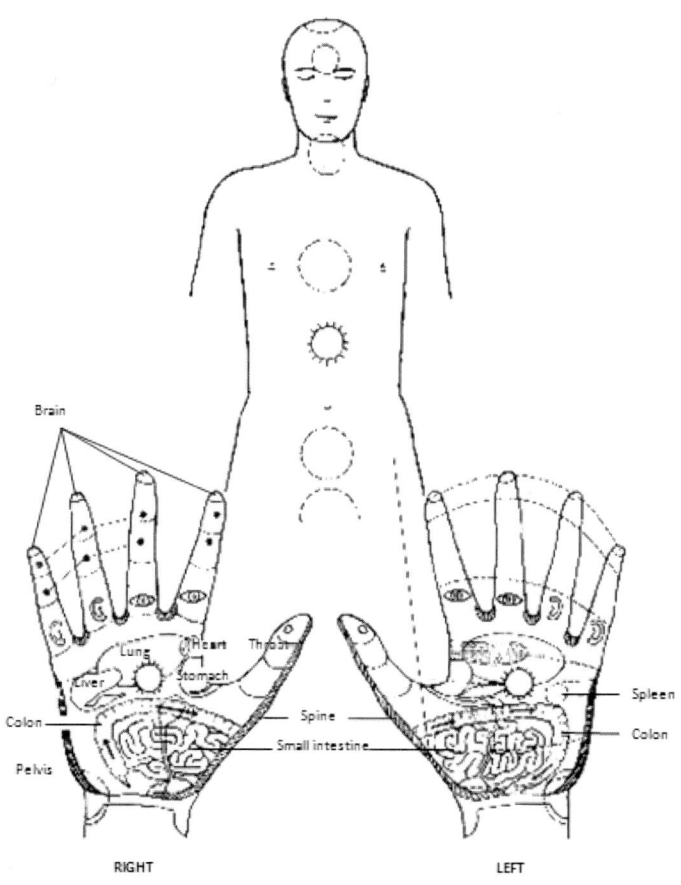

# 3. MEDITATION METHODS

There are plenty of books that suggest a spiritual seeker should start with meditation exercises. Such meditations are then usually a purely mental exercise, because the practitioner has not yet learned or recognized to experience his whole body as a resonance chamber for the unlimited energy of happiness.

Therefore, the previous chapters were very important, in order for us to understand that a comprehensive transformation must involve our whole being. All the more sweet and ripe the fruits of happiness will be, that we can then harvest by meditation methods.

While our feelings are related to certain areas of the body, our thoughts are very strongly located in our head. In meditation we will thus have the task to realize that our thoughts and the connected mind also represent a part of our being, but that we still are more than the sum of our thoughts and the associated attitudes and views.

*Stopping the flow of thoughts*

Some time ago I read the advertising slogan of a large german company: "We never stop thinking." This made me smile, because this is exactly what represents the biggest obstacle on the way to our unlimited happiness – the thinking. As useful as the mind may be in scientific activity and the innovation of new technologies or just for solving some trivial everyday affairs; the constant thought processes hinder the accumulation of biophotons.

In order to ignite the flame of happiness behind our forehead and under our crown, a certain concentration of high-frequency biophotons is required at specific locations of our brain. The fact that such accumulation occurs spontaneously, is unlikely because of the constant thought process that disperses the bioplasma energy in the mind. Therefore, we need methods that help us in the accumulation of biophotons. We need sparks and tinder to ignite the flame in our pituitary and pineal glands.

# SILENT MEDITATION

In the methods learnt, we have always "done" something. Meditation is the exact opposite of that, when we meditate, we do nothing at all. We just let happen. In meditation we turn our attention inward.

During silent meditation we assume internally the attitude of a detatched observer. We perceive the emotions that we feel and the thoughts that we think, but we do not want to identify ourselves with them. We try to keep a small inner distance to our feelings and thoughts. We are simply observing. This in itself is a pleasant experience, if we find that we are more than our feelings and thoughts with which we constantly identify ourselves.

We are in a state of pure consciousness that exists independently of feelings and thoughts. If this pure consciousness manifests itself within us, we will penetrate to the true and eternal core of our our lifes.

*Gain Distance*

We will catch ourselves again and again in how we jump during silent meditation on to the train of our thoughts and get familiar with them.

The essential practice of silent meditation consists of avoiding this popping up on the train of thoughts automatically and to be able to not identify ourselves with them more and more often and to realise that our thought apparatus, our mind, has become independent from us and has supplied us with some kind of substitute identity.

The silent meditation is therefore first of all the medium to enable us to take on a detached attitude towards our thoughts and feelings – become an uninvolved observer.

This is an essential prerequisite for the manifestation

of a fully conscious and liberated state of being in us. On the quantum level this means that we, by the distance and observation of our feelings and thoughts, identify ourselves with photons of a higher frequency and in this way with a higher energy. Pure consciousness is composed of photons of higher frequency and higher energy than the photons that constitute our thoughts.

*Concentrating the life energy by „not-doing"*

The meditation has the consequence that a focus – a concentration – of our life energy takes place in our body. And especially in our brain an ever stronger energy field ist built up which is formed through high energy photons of a high frequency and high internal order. Meditation helps us to enrich a high-energy coherent quantum field inside of us.

We literally don't need to do anything ourselves in meditation in order for the concentrated energy field of pure consciousness to form inside of us. This happens completely on its own, because photons of high frequency and thus high energy are ubiquitous and our body matter – namely the electrons – want to automatically assume a higher degree of order, if we do not stop them through our incessant bustle.

In meditation – in „non-action" - we are beginning to recognise that our true nature and being are not relying on doing something constantly in order to get access to the ubiquitous and inexhaustible photon field.

Before somebody deals with meditation, he is constantly distracted and does not realise that he bears the access to the source of his life, which guarantees him fulfillment, joy and happiness, already within himself.

We have in each of the  trillions  of cells in our body in the form of DNA, optimal receiving antennas, with which we can absorb the photon field of life and happiness in us. If we do not constantly hinder our body through our mental activities to assume an optimal energy state, we will continue to manifest such a state of happiness within us.

The silent meditation helps us to overcome the dominance of our mental activities and enables us to let the harmonious, coherent photon field take place in our system. The constant „chatter" of our mind is restrained with the increase of the high-energy photon field. So the mind becomes a tool again which we use if needed – but if it is not necessary to think about something and there is nothing to decide, we can just take on our natural state of being, which is formed by the happy stream of a high-energy photon field.

*The happy spark ignites*

The high-energy photons are waiting in the gaps between the thoughts to be discovered by us. Here, in the short and important absence of a thought  a  stronger awareness independent from our mind can mature.

When we exhale deeply in the silent meditation and let go inside, the first happy sparks can flare up in the gap between two thoughts. The nerve tissue of the brain is the flammable tinder. At first, after having trained ourselves in the silent meditation for a while, we will be able to perceive individual small happy sparks behind our forehead, between the eyebrows – a pleasant tingle. Once our body's own biophoton field has been sufficiently unfolded and released by transformation, we will perceive these happy sparks more often in the silent meditation. Then there will ripen a small happy flame, which we can stir up and also enjoy in silent meditation. The flame develops inside the head, anatomically seen at the location of the pituitary gland. From there it will be getting stronger and reaches above a certain bioplasma concentration in the epiphysis (pineal gland) which is at the centre of the skull. If a certain threshold is reached, then the flame ignites like a glistening cutting torch and cannot be extinguished any more. This is the enlightenment.

*What „Enlightenment" means*

When enlightenment happens, the inner light patterns of a part of our electrons get so strongly focused that they dissolve, i.e the contained photon energy and information is able to go into the hyperspace. It is a redemption process.

in which the energy that was bound in the material electrons is released and can return to the place where it came from. Between the electrons that have reached this highest concentrated condition at the apex center and for the remaining electrons whose inner photon energy is not yet as highly concentrated, there is, however, still a strong interaction. Energy rich photons get exchanged between the electrons and this is how the happiness-flow starts.

When this lucky flame blazes through the whole body, in principle a state can be achieved, in which all electrons reach the highest photon concentration. Then, the body is immortal and has obtained all degrees of freedom – salvation and physical immortality – and the possiblity to bring the whole body to this state and ascend into the hyperspace, from which comes all the energy that has manifested itself as matter in the outer time space – our universe.

*It takes Practice and Patience*

With the body-oriented transformation methods that were described in the previous chapters, we can release our vital life energy. Then, it will not be difficult for us, after some practicing of silent meditation, to kindle the stream of happiness that waits between our thoughts.

There are some people, who have been meditating for years and the flame does not want to ignite. Here, not enough has been done, to solve the energy blockades that have manifested themselves in the body, through body-oriented methods and to resolve them by transformation and release the life energy.

Let us imagine, we have no matches and no lighter to start a fire. Who among us could still light a fire in the way primitive men were capable of? It takes a little spark and some highly flammable material.

Whoever succeeds once to perceive and foment the happy flame in silent meditation, will be able to assume this pleasant state again and again through this exercise. The happy flame – consisting of energy-rich biophotons – will be able to increase in size and our inner awareness ability will grow and expand along with it.

## SILENT MEDITATION:

The starting position: Outwardly, we take on a posture that allows our bioplasma energy to circulate freely and undisturbed in our body. We can sit in a chair, our back straight, just like it has been described in chapter 1, exercise 1 (page 26). If you like, you can of course also sit in the yoga- or heel-seat on the floor. A straight posture of the spine is important, so that our energy centres are aligned vertically one above the other in this meditation, in order to optimize the energy flow and the intake and movement of Eta-particles, which always come vertically from above (our body can convert a part of the gravitational quantum – I call them eta-particles – into biophotons; find more details on page 78f. and in my book „The Ancient Word – The Physics of God").

For some people it is easier in the beginning to adapt to a relaxed upright posture, by leaning against the back of a chair. This is fine. The exercise is not about forcing our body into an unusual posture, but instead we want to gently and without the use of force achieve a pleasant state of being.

Conscious breathing serves as a basis for silent meditation as well. We breathe harmoniously and slowly in and out and make sure to reach the abdomen as well with our breath, as it was described in the breathing exercises in chapter 1.

> We breathe deeply and harmoniously and relax and let go.

> We close our eyes during silent meditation and let ourselves not be distracted by outside noises.

> We focus our attention inwards, but take the attitude of an indifferent observer towards our feelings and thoughts.

> We concentrate ourselves on to the gaps between our thoughts and during the deep breathing we let go of everything – right here is, where the lucky sparks are waiting for us.

> Between the eyebrows will gradually ignite a small happy flame. By further release and expansion of the

thought gaps, it will grow, until a strong, glistening flame of light becomes of it. If this flame continues to grow and reaches the apex of our head, it can be so bright that it outshines all thoughts. Now, we are no longer slaves to our mind, but can use it according to our will.

> A perpetuous happiness flow gets underway, of which we cannot get rid of anymore. Our being and our nature are flooded more and more by love and happiness. We feel completely alive and refresehed.

Our energy system can now go through an accelerated process of transformation. We get a deeper access to our soul and it is no longer difficult for us to remember earlier incarnations with the help of appropriate methods.

The silent meditation is the most important and crucial step on the way to the development of our happiness potential, because only in practicing the silent meditation, are we able to calm our thought process and eventually learn to switch it on and off at our own discretion.  This is precisely the condition by which the lucky current can be set in motion, by activating the energy centres in our head and  by igniting the happy flame.

Whenever we have time to ourselves, we can enter this state and enjoy the happiness flood that then ripples through our bodies from head to toe.

# MIRROR MEDITATION

When I spent some vacaction time in the winter of 1984/85 on the Canary Island La Gomera, I started with a mirror meditation one evening. It was already dark and I looked at my reflection in the mirror by candellight and fixed a point between the eybrows. I tried to blik as little as possible with my eyes – and suddenly I saw another face in the mirror. It was the face of an older man. A light shudder trickled down my spine. For the first time, I looked into the face of one of my former incarnations.

That evening a gate flung open in my soul, which should not be closed again. It was the beginning of an awakening of my soul. At night the inner psychic space that had been unlocked through the mirror meditation, was opened even further. In dreams more details of the previous life came into my consciousness.

Before I started with the mirror meditation, I had fueled my energy system for some time with body oriented methods and silent meditation. As a result, I was given a deep access to my soul history.

*Performing the exercise*

In the mirror meditation one simply sits upright and comfortable in front of a mirror and looks at the reflection of ones own face. The room is slightly darkened and next to the mirror two candles can be placed. The eyes stare in the mirror and fix a certain point in the mirror image. Unconscious soul information can come to the surface like this and the face can change. Initially, the eyes will quickly water, but with some practice, you will be able to stare into the mirror without blinking. As with other meditations emotional showers may trickle through the body. Whenever it tingles like this, the body's electrons exchange light particles among themselves and previously unknown information is passed over to the whole of the electrons. Don't forget deep and conscious breathing.

**Effects:** When we get a deeper access to our soul through the mirror meditation, old inner images and feelings are revealed to us as a consequence. Possibly, intense dreams may follow in which we process the flood of intra-psychic forces that break free.

It is generally very useful to remember what we have dreamt after waking up. The processing can be continued in the waking consciousness and with time many individual pieces of information can be put together in a soul-mosaic and we progressively receive an overview of our soul history.

## QUANTUM MEDITATION

A recommendation to anyone who wants to practice this form of meditation is: to read my book: The Ancient Word - The Physics of God.

It provides an overview of the quantum sea surrounding us and the various forms of energy contained therein, such as spacial structure energy and light energy, eta particles and photons.

Yet, a short overview will also be procured here about the various forms of energy and their expression as well as their significance for our spiritual transformation.

*The Eta-Particles*

From God – the hyperspace source ELI – eta-particles emerge which span not only the hyperspace itself, but also all other realms that came out of the hyperspace. In our universe, the outer space time is spanned by Eta-particles which may crystallise into quantum structure areas. In addition, new Eta-particles are constantly flowing into our universe from the hyperspace.

These Eta-particles follow the course of the gravitational field. So, they always fly to where matter is already in the room. On the surface of the earth, where we live, these Eta-particles always come from above – that is the preferred direction to the hyperspace. These Eta-particles rain down on us and they are the reason that we are pressed towards the earth. They are forming the quantum of gravity.

All good things come from above – most Eta-particles raining down on us, penetrate us freely and fly on in the direction of the centre of the earth. However, some of them bounce off the atoms of our body and are reflected back to the hyperspace. Others are not reflected in our body matter, but swirl on annular molecular structures – e.g. in the nucleic bridges of the DNA in our cells – and in this way connect together photons from the quantum sea into our organism. These biophotons control the metabolism and life process in our cells and care for generating electromagnetic fields in the nerve-tissue that make up our feelings, thoughts and our happy flame.

*Exercises for the Eta-Energy*

The first exercise for the quantum meditation is therefore dedicated to the Eta-particles, since they contribute to the preservation of our vitality and the development of our consciousness.

In all the exercises described below, we assume the inner attitude of an uninvolved observer, which was described earlier in the practice of the silent meditation at the beginning of this chapter. We breathe calmly and deeply in and out.

Standing up exercise to receive Eta-Particles: In Greek the letter Eta is written as H. We stand upright, our feet are parallel to each other with about a foot distance in between. Our arms are stretched upwards parallel. The palms face upwards and the hands are about a foot apart as well. We form the shape of the letter Eta:

We look our forward during this meditation, but can then close the eye lids. In this exercise we get charged stronger than usual with the divine power of the eta particles.

We can hold this position as long as it is not difficult for us and thereby accumulate free hyperspace energy inside of us.

**Exercise to receive eta-particles lying down:** We can take the same posture while lying down comfortably. Legs and arms are parallel, feet and hands about a foot apart. The arms are stretched out backwards while lying on the floor, palms facing up.

*Exercises concerning Chi-Energy*

The field lines of electrostatic fields are radially symmetrical. They radiate in all directions or are running together to a point from all directions. In the Original-Word-Theory such star shaped radiating fields are referred to as Chi.

**Standing up exercise for the activation of chi-energy:** The Greek letter Chi is written as X. We stand with our legs slightly straddled. The feet are about a meter apart. The arms are stretched upwards and the hands are also a few feet apart.

The exercise by lying down to receive Chi-Energy: This exercise can be done lying down. While lying on the floor, we spread the legs and arms to the sides – hands and feet are each about a meter apart.

This exercise connects our consciousness with all directions – with the world as a whole.

*Exercises concerning the Phi-Energy*

The field lines of magnetic fields are self-contained and therefore more or less circular. In the Ancient-Word-Theory, such fields, which close in on themselves are referred to as Phi.

**Exercise 1 for the activating of Phi-Energy:** The Greek letter Phi is written as Φ. We stand upright. Feet together and pointing straight ahead.The arms form a circle, whith the elbows pointing outwards laterally and the hands are above the body on the belly button.

Exercise 2 for receiving Phi-Energy: Lying down on the floor, we stretch our legs out parallel, so that the feet are touching. The arms form a circle again, with the elbows pointing outwards laterally and the hands resting one above the other on the belly button.

In this exercise we can let the energy circulate in our body.

*Exercises concerning the Theta-Energy*

Out of the structural flow of Eta, Chi and Phi, the Theta vortices may form. One can assume that our universe emerged out of a theta-vortex, which was fueled in hyperspace. The elementary constituents of matter, the electrons and positrons can be represented as theta vortices. Theta-vortices play an important role in the provision of vital life energy in the form of biophotons in biological structures.

Our vitality and joy of life are obtained from theta-vortices. In the unfolding of the human energy system, large theta vortices form the main energy centres also known as chakras in wisdom teachings. The properties and functions of these chakras we will come to this in the next chapter.

**Standing up exercise for the activation of Theta Energy:** The Greek letter Theta is written as Θ. We stand straight. Our feet are closed and pointing straight ahead. The arms form a circle, whereas the elbows point outwards laterally. The palms meet over the head and lie on each other. The inner surfaces of the hands can be showing up or down.

Exercise lying down for the receiving of Theta-Energy: The same posture may also be taken lying down. We stretch the legs out parallel, so that the feet are touching.

The arms form a circle again, with the elbows at the sides facing outwards and the hands meet behind the head.

## ELI MEDITATION

ELI is the source of all energy in the universe – Energy, Love and Information. There is nothing that could make us happier than to connect with this source. In the hyperspace ELI radiates high energy eta-particles in all directions. The higher eta-particle energies we are capable of attaching to us, the more the photon gas inside our electrons can pool to photons with high frequency. And thus we can receive more and more biophotons, to realize our happiness potential. Therefore, we give all the glory to ELI, and connect with ELI in a standing up exercise.

Lambda-Theta, omnipotence, Alpha-Omega and omnipresence merge in this icon for ELI. I am the A (Alpha) and the O (Omega) the Beginning and the End.

**Standing up exercise to connect with ELI:** We stand upright, our feet are parallel and about fiftiy centimeters apart.

> Our arms, hands and fingertips are stretched upwards, with the palms touching symmetrically as in the attitude of prayer. In this posture we have aligned every fiber of our being to ELI.

> After a while, our hands make contact so that they are symmetrically touching at the palms, vertically downwards, first to the level of our forehead and remain in this position for a little while.

> Then we lead the hands further down to the level of the throat and remain in this position also for some time.

> Finally, we take the hands down to the middle of our chest and remain in this position.

We are intimately connected to ELI, the ubiquitous and all-encompassing energy, love and information.

*Visual ELI Meditation*

The symbol for ELI, the Lambda-Theta and the Alpha-Omega, can also be comtemplated in a silent meditation. Since this symbol represents the omnipotence and omnipresence in an appropriate way, we are able to connect with ELI through a silent contemplation of it.

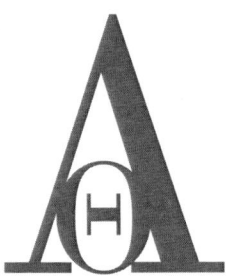

My personal experience with ELI is one of a deep and trusting relationship. For me,

ELI is more than an impersonal energy and power, in which I can immerse with my consciousness. ELI flows through and floods everything there is – but ELI is more than his creation. ELI is the Ancient Word, and from this primoridal word all vibrations – sounds – emerged.

ELI is also a personal god. ELI is a being. ELI is a person. ELI can even manifest in physical form. The one and eternal god, ELI has many names.

For me personally, my access to god opens up not only through meditation, but also through prayer and the autonomous celebration of the Holy Communion and other Christian Sacraments. But to this theme range I would like to dedicate an entire book of its own. I cannot contribute my personal relationship with god as a method of spiritual transformation here.


## ANCIENT WORD MEDITATION

In the Ancient-Word-Theory, the primal word matrix forms a symmetrical arrangement of the structure of quantized fluxes, from which emerge all spatio-temporal structures and thus all of our physical, mental and spiritual realms.

The contemplation of the Ancient-Word-Matrix imparts a strong connection to ELI and all energies that emerge from ELI.

The looking at of the ancient word matrix is highly invigorating. It reminds us of the entirety of the omnipresent quantum sea, in which we all swim.

$$X \ A \ \Theta \ \Omega \ \Phi$$

$$A \ \Phi \ H \ X \ \Omega$$

$$\Theta \ H \ \mathring{A} \ H \ \Theta$$

$$\Omega \ X \ H \ \Phi \ A$$

$$\Phi \ \Omega \ \Theta \ A \ X$$

In the centre of the Ancient Word Matrix is ELI, represented by the Lambda-Theta and Alpha-Omega symbol. ELI radiates eta-particles in all four dimensions of the hyperspace, which is spread out through this. From two mutually perpendicular eta particles Chi- and Phi-energies are formed and therefore photons as well. Through this, the inner region of the light filled hyperspace is stretched out – the heaven.

From Eta-, Chi- and Phi-energies Theta-Vortices are formed. These Theta-Vortices form spatiotemporal structures, in which our lives are shaped. The lower theta-vortex represents our universe, the outer space-time, the here and now. The upper theta-vortices represents the inner space-time, the soul landscapes, the beyond. The two lateral theta-vortex form the polar charged electrons and positrons and thus the basic building blocks of all matter and also the individual intra-psychic memory contents. The spatio temporal character of the theta-vortex, in each of which exists a time-like transition dimension, is represented by the alphas and omegas.

# 4. EARLIER INCARNATIONS

## HIDDEN GIFTS AND ANCIENT BURDENS

Anyone who enters into an intense spiritual transformation process, cannot avoid the subject of reincarnation and the conscious confrontation with one's own past lives sooner or later.

In my book The Ancient Word – The Physics of God, I have designed a quantum physical model of the human soul, from which the individual memory contents of a person is stored in a part of the human body

– in the essence electrons. Some particle-models in physics stress indeed that electrons have an individual memory and this information does not get lost even after the physical death of a living being because electrons have, in theory, an infinite life time. The essence electrons of a living being leave the body at death, stay together further on as a diluted part of the abandoned body and represent the immortal soul of a creature. In a reincarnation a new body crystallizes around the essence electrons.

During the physical life phase, the essence electrons stick preferably to the regions of the body where there is the least change through metabolic processes or cell neoplasms.This is the part, where the cells of the central nervous system are located – that is, the brain, the spinal cord and the nervous tissue.

Since the essence electrons form a small fraction only compared to the whole of the body matter, the information about earlier incarnations contained in the essence electrons is at first not directly accessible to the consciousness – they form in their entirety the individual subconsciousness of a person.

Through spiritual transformation methods we can elicit the stored information from the essence electrons and make it accessible to the consciousness.

## Resolve Traumas of the Past

The recollection of earlier incarnations is not about the rediscovery of famous historical persons or about eliciting extraneous details from the inexhaustible reservoir of information of the essence electrons.

Rather, it is important to become aware again of traumatic experiences from earlier lives because these still prevent us from unfolding our full happiness potential today. Traumatic experiences from previous incarnations block us just as much as similar experiences that happened in this life.

In order to live freely and in the present,

we also need a deeper conscious access to our spiritual part. Those who do not care about the mastering and processing of their legacy from the past with appropriate methods, will be limited by it in the development of his happiness potential in the now. It is then as if one drags a heavy weight chained to the foot behind oneself or even as if one is running around with a millstone around one's neck.

### The Endless Loop of Recurring Manifestations

The repetition of the repetition. Many people believe that they experience how they live now for the first time, but they do not realize that they play an old record over again and again. As long as we are not aware of our old patterns and affinities, they will keep trying to manifest themselves a new over and over again. As multi-dimensional beings, we ourselves are a bridge between spirit and matter. What is stored in the memory banks of our essence electrons in light patterns, is the process of interaction between them and the rest of our body matter which is to be manifested again.

Whenever I had created through a meditation, for example the mirror meditation, a new access to an earlier incarnation that had been unknown to me so far, I felt a shiver going down my spine. It was mildly scary to me, since the boundary between the subconscious and the conscious had been opened. However, it is not surprising that there were shivers running down my back, because in the spine also runs a major nerve cord that connects the brain with all areas of the body and there, in the central nervous system, most of the essence electrons are located. These somewhat eerie sensations are related to the fact that in the moment of the remembrance-chills, information that was only stored in the essence electrons before this, is now passed on to the totality of the body forming eletrons.

As a consequence, the conscious processing of the recollected old experiences began. We are now confronted with different feelings – such as fear, pain, despair. But we can also remember beautiful experiences that we bring in connection with a loved one who is close to us.

I will remember the enormous rise of vitality and joy of life, which I experienced in the beginning of 1986 when I recalled the violent death I had suffered about 3000 years ago in Egypt. All the pain of that death experience swept through my body. It was anything but pleasant and some parts of my body were really quite sore, but the old trauma melted away and after that I felt more free and more alive than ever before in this lifetime.

You can say that the conscious access to past lifes and the trauma experienced therein, initially represents a psychich challenge which needs to be processed but, after going through such a remembrance and transformation process, one has achieved a significantly greater freedom and vitality. Death is stuck in the bones in all of us.

Through the conscious transforming of such an old shock of events, we liberate ourselves from karmic burdens. We should be aware that our subconscious repeatedly tries to manifest old experiences from the past in the present again in the form of subtle electromagnetic fields of the essence electrons. With the information that they carry collectively, they generate electromagnetic fields – photon fields -  which create an affinity to the repetition of the trauma suffered. Each trauma that lies dormant in our subconscious is like a time bomb that can blow up at ay time of our lives, which then catches up with us in the form of a fatality.

The only alternative to escape such fate-shocks, is the conscious and deliberate confrontation and processing in a spiritual transformation process, it can be initiated by the presented methods.

If we want to attain liberation from such blockages from previous incarnations, we will also need to engage in appropriate methods that give us a conscious access to such old information. With the mirror meditation we have already learnt one way in which we can delve into the depths of our souls. Another method – the introspection during the guided recall – will be explained below.

# INTROSPECTION AND GUIDED RECALL

It makes sense to use this method only once we have already gained some experience with the earlier described breathing techniques, relaxation and letting-go exercises as well as the body-oriented stretching and meditation methods.

**Introspection exercise in lying down:** This exercise can only be carried out alone in limitation. It is better to do it with a partner. One person goes into the introspection and the other person is accompanying the guided recall.

It makes sense to perform an introspection with recall while lying down because at the beginning we perform a deep relaxation, as described in Chapter 1, page 33 ff.

Lie down comfortably on a firm couch or on a blanket on the ground and cover ourselves with a blanket. We are not letting ourselves be distracted from external noises and direct our entire attention inward.

1.    **Deep Relaxation:** The accompanying person sits down on a chair next to the person lying down and gives instructions for the deep relaxation. For this purpose the text of the deep relaxation (you form) can be used.

2.   **Guided Recall:** After the deep relaxation the accompanying person begins with the recall. During this we move with our consciousness into the past. The guided person can say something to the accompanying

person at each time station, if they want to, especially if they are perceiving unpleasant feelings.

Suppose the person lying down is 40 years old, then the accompanying person may initiate the recalling with the following words:

> "Remember the past events of your life. If you want to say something that you have experienced, just talk about it."

> "You are 30 years old now. Can you perceive something?" (The guided person says something or half a minute break).

> "Now, you are 20 years old. Can you perceive something?" (The guided person says something or half a minute break).

> "Now, you are 15 years old. Can you perceive something?" (The guided person says something or half a minute break).

> "You are ten years old now. Can you perceive something?" (The guided person says something or half a minute break).

> "You are five years old now. Can you perceive something?" (The guided person says something or half a minute break).

> "You are a toddler now. Can you perceive something?" (The guided person says something or half a minute break)

94

> "You are a baby now. Can you perceive something?" (The guided person says something or half a minute break).

> "You are born now. Can you perceive something?" (The guided person says something or half a minute break).

> "You are born now. Can you perceive something?" (The guided person says something or half a minute break).

**Interjection Remark:** The recall does not necessarely have to result in a past life. If the guided person has to look at some event in this life, for example in their youth or childhood and finds intense feelings there, one can stay in this time range during the introspection and the guided person can talk all about what they experienced there, in order to process later what happened at this time.

The accompanying person should not make any suggestive remarks but as far as possbile only ask questions. If the guided person describes a negative feeling, the accompanying person can ask for example: "Where did this happen?" or "How did your father or your mother react?" Unpleasant feelings mainly remain stored in reference to situations in the family, at shool or in a relationship.

If an unpleasant feeling appears, for example fear, pain, sadness or anger, then the guided person can talk all about it, take a deep breath and let go of the emotion and transform it.

The guiding person can support the person doing the recall in the processing of unpleasant feelings or perceived pain with the following words, for example: "Just breathe deeply and let go of the pain (or the fear, anger, sadness)."

If no situations need to be looked at in this life who left behind a trauma, we go further back in time. The accompanying person then continues with the words:

> "It is now 1950. Can you perceive something?" (The guided person says something or half a minute break).

> "It is now 1940. Can you perceive something?" (The guided person says something or half a minute break).

One can also undertake larger steps into the past or deliberately seek a specific historic site or land.

> "We are now in the year 1800. Can you perceive something?" (The guided person says something or half a minute break).

> "We are now in the year 1700. Can you perceive something?" (The guided person says something or half a minute break).

> "We are now in the year 1600. Can you perceive something?" (The guided person says something or half a minute break).

With these formulations you can always go further back in time. A retrospection can also span several millenia or even further back to long lost cultures like Atlantis, but first of all you shoud illuminate the recent past. This will not happen in one sitting, but is a realization and transformation process which stretches over a longer period of time.

Initially, it is not important to which exact past time the recall leads. The crucial fact is, that the guided person has a perception, which they cannot assign to events from this life. Here you can focus on the perceived scene.

It is also very individual how guided back persons perceive past events. Some behold inner images that they only have to tell, but more important than any internal films are authentic feelings that appear during introspection. If it is a question of unpleasant emotions such as fear, anger or pain, there is an energetic blockage which is emanating from the emotion and we want to dissolve these in order to augment the hap piness currently inside of us. The primary goal of the looking inward is to solve internal blockages of our souls and to process traumatic experiences and not to talk about any petty details which have no relation to the current emotional state of the guided person.

Narrow down the Memory precisely: If the guided person approaches an unpleasant feeling or pain, it makes sense to look at the context or the scene in detail:

> "Can you see where you are now? Describe the location or the room you are in."

> "Can you see who is there?"

> "What exactly happened?"

> "How did you get into this situation?"

It is possible that a person can locate a pain exactly in the body during introspection and recalls for example that a knife was rammed into their belly or chest or that they were beheaded. If such memories are coming up, it is very helpful to breathe into the pain and release it. This may cause the guided person to cry. The accompanying partner should then comfort them. It is advisable to keep tissues ready to be able to wipe away any tears. If a spot on the body is hurting, the guided person may also put her hands there.

After half an hour to one hour a scene should be sufficently illuminated so that we can go back on the path to the present.

**The return back to the present:** An introspection should not be stopped abruptly. Although, the method described here takes place with the guide person completely conscious, but nevertheless, they may have opened up sensitive intrapsychic areas and as gently and carefully as we have approached these places, we also want to leave them behind us and move on.

We should use all of the love and power of thoughts at our disposal in order to connect the accessible and opened soul area with the waking consciousness. On the way back to the present, the accompanying person can use the following phrases, depending on how far back we have looked, for example:

> "We are now in the year 1600." (Ten seconds pause)

> "We are now in the year 1700." (Ten seconds pause)

> "We are now in the year 1800." (Ten seconds pause)

> "We are now in the year 1900." (Ten seconds pause)

> "We are now in the year 1950." (Ten seconds pause)

> "Now you are in the belly of your mother." (Ten seconds pause)
> "You are now being born." (Ten seconds pause)
> "You are now a baby." (Ten seconds pause)
> "You are now five years old." (Ten seconds pause)
> "You are now ten years old." (Ten seconds pause)
> "You are now 20 years old." (Ten seconds pause)
> "You are now 30 years old." (Ten seconds pause)
> "You are now 40 years old." (Ten seconds pause)
> 'You are back in the present. You can open your eyes again."

The guided person should take some time and remain lying before getting up again and before life goes on in the present, somewhat more liberated and happier.

**Aftereffects:** If we have remembered a traumatizing event by looking inside, such as a severe physical or psychological injury or a violent death, the physical and psychological processing of the memory is not yet completed with the introspection. In the days that follow, certain parts of the body will be affected by the old injury, which may cause pain or violent emotions which will flow through our body. It may also occur that they have intense dreams afterwards, in which they process their memories further on a spiritual level.

In the transformation process which follows an introspection, the previously learnt breathing techniques and the body-oriented methods will be of help to us, to integrate the memories and to resolve the associated blockages in our energy system. It is also advisable to speak with people we trust and who have developped a spiritual awareness themselves, about the experience and thus to process it further.


*Recalls under Hypnosis*

There are reincarnation therapists who trace their clients previous lifes under hypnosis. Although the information obtained is often quite spectacular, because a large volume of information is collected here, the guided person has only a small benefit from it for their own spiritual transformation because they rarely remember, after waking up from the state of hypnosis, what they saw i.e. perceived during the recall. I am therefore not sympathatic to recalls under hypnosis and prefer to enable people to get a conscious access to the past of their souls in order for them to consciously process the experience and in this way solve the associated loads and energy blockades.

# 5. ENERGY CENTRES AND QUANTUM HEALING

## THE ENERGY CENTRES – CHAKRAS

Anyone who has gained a certain amount of experiences with spiritual tansformation methods over a period of time, will notice, after a while, that there are paticular areas of the body where life energy is concentrated. In addition to the energy channels, the so called acupuncture

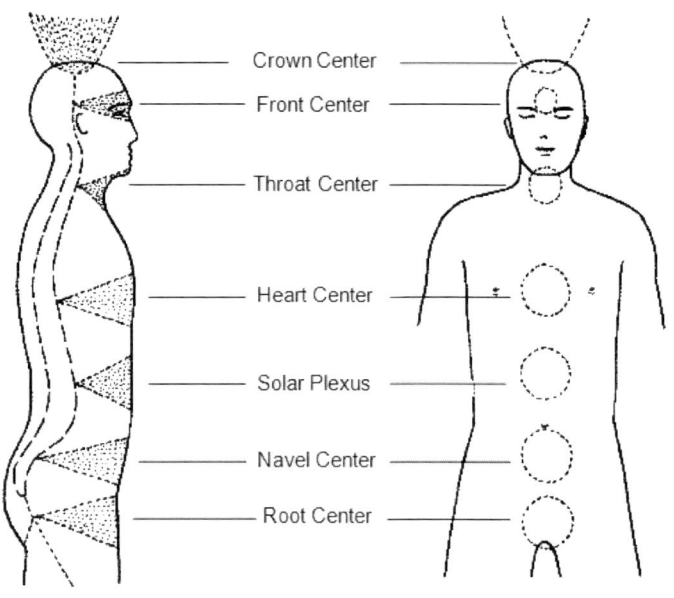

Crown Center

Front Center

Throat Center

Heart Center

Solar Plexus

Navel Center

Root Center

meridians, which are known from traditional chinese medicine and with which we have dealt in connection to the stretching exercises, there exist seven main energy centres in the human body in which the vital energy of the quantum biophotons are swirled and distributed all over the body. In eastern teachings they are called chakras. The illustration above shows a side and a front view of the energy centres.

There are the root and navel centre, the solar plexus, the heart, the throat, the front centre or third eye and the crown centre. The energy whirl of the chakras unfolds from the spine to the front of the body. From the crown center the radiation goes upwards to the skull.

*Shifted vertebrae restrict the flow of energy*

In order for the energy channels to develop between the centres, not only is the opening of the acupuncture meridians of importance but also an upright posture where the spine is not distorted.

We have put great importance on some exercises, especially on silent meditation and on an upright posture, so that the spine is straight and no shifts between the individual vertebrae occur; which may otherwise cause a jam in the energy flow of the essence electrons. In many people there are shifts between certain vertebrae, partly due to poor posture in childhood and in youth during this life, partly due to traumas developped in earlier lives and formed again in an early stage of physical development in this lifetime. Such disturbances in the spine can be corrected by awareness of having the correct posture or through appropriate chiropractic treatment.

*Tasks of the Chakras*

Each of the seven main energy centres has special tasks for the organization of life processes.

## 1. Root Centre

**Healthy Function:** The root centre is located in the groin between the anus and the genitals as well as at the end of the coccyx. The main frequency range of biophotons here is the colour red (in the range of visible light) and, as with all other centres, in multiple frequency values of the colour. The root chakra's mission is to connect the body to the earth (grounding) and to convey a harmonious relationship with matter.

**Disturbed Function:** A weekened or severely blocked root center points to the storage of negative feelings such as existencial anxiety or fear to loose the ground under ones feet. Often this results in difficulties in meeting one's own material needs, such as a troubled relationship with money or problems to earn one's own livelihood; also the inclination not to allow any benefits or positive things to oneself or others. Also, neglect on a physical level, lacking hygiene or poor clothing, a bad and unbalanced diet are signs of a root centre with hypofunction. A strong disturbance of the function of the root chakra can also lead to a muffled energy flow of bioplasma through the legs to the feet. Blockades then often sit on the inner side of the thighs above the knee, in the knee itself and in the ankles.

## 2. Navel Centre

**Healthy Function:** The navel centre is located a few inches below the belly button. The frequency of the exchanged photons corresponds to the colour orange. The navel centre controls the function of the sexual glands, ie ovaries, prostate and testicles. The navel chakra is also the reservoir for bioplasma, ie for life energy.

**Disturbed Function:** Pent-up unexpressed emotions, such as anger, lead to a disturbance of the navel centre. Many individual and interpersonal problems have their starting point here, for example sexual difficulties or emotional dependencies, menstrual problems, jealousy, dislike of one's own body, lack of self-esteem. But also excessive sexual expression leads to a weakening of the navel centre and thus as a result to the lowering of vitality and an acceleration of the aging processes.

## 3. Solar Plexus

**Healthy Function:** The solar plexus is about a hand's breadth above the belly button. The main colour of the light particles is yellow. This energy centre is related to the pancreas. In the solar plexus the life energy that is stored in the navel centre gets transported to the outside.

In the body the utilisation and the excretion of metabolic wastes (digestion) are controlled by the solar plexus.

**Disturbed Function:** Aggression and fighting are the downsides of an imbalanced solar plexus. Thus, the creative life energy flows destructively to the outside. Also exaggerated pursuits of power and disregard of the free will of others are an expression of an imbalanced solar plexus function. If the working of the solar plexus is strongly reduced, it is due to the repressed feelings of helplessness, passivity, victim attitudes or lack of assertiveness stored here.

4. Heart Centre

**Healthy Function:** In the heart centre the electrons exchange predominantly green light particles of the visible light range. The heart centre corresponds with the thymus gland, the function of which is important for the body's immune system and the defense against viruses and other pathogens. In the interpersonal realm the heart centre conveys loving encounters with other people and generally an attitude determined and supported by love toward all beings and all of creation.

The heart centre is of central importance for the energy system of man, since it is located exactly in the middle of the seven centres of the energy channel. The heart centre therefore mediates between the three lower, material-oriented energy centres and the top three, mentally oriented ones.

**Disturbed Function:** In a troubled heart centre inferior feelings, such as distrust and hate towards oneself and others and also sadness, loneliness, desolation and lack of love can be found. Even the widespread burnout syndrome is associated with a disturbed heart centre. There are problems with meeting other people and living things with love and openness. Also the ability to accept love from the outside, from other people stagnates due to a disturbed heart centre. Through closed hearts people cause a lot of suffering to each other because the ability to feel compassion is then lost.

A strong blockage of the heart centre can result, if there are other risk factors present, in problems such as heart attacks and lung cancer.

## 5. Throat Centre

**Healthy Function:** The preferred colour in the area of the throat centre is turquoise. Physically the throat center is related to the thyroid gland. Also, all respiratory organs are controlled by both the throat centre and the heart centre. Mentally, the throat centre is responsible for a clear verbal communication. The ability of free and uninhibited utterance and self-presentation to the outside are some of the qualities of this energy centre.

**Disturbed Function:** If the throat centre is not fully opened, a person will have difficulties in expressing clearly their needs, feelings and perceptions to the outside. The fear of showing oneself to other people and to communicate, shyness and stage fright are among the weaknesses of an underdevelopped throat centre – the proverbial lump in the neck is one also and to swallow and choke down feelings is a nother mechanism that leads to a blockage of the throat chakra.

## 6. Front Centre

Healthy Function: The front centre, also called the third eye, is located approximately between the eyebrows and it corresponds on the visible light range  with the colour dark blue. The pituitary gland is on the endocrine level associated with the front centre. Here is the seat of creativity, ingenuity, virtuosity and vision. Once the front centre is activated there will be a clarification of consciousness and the electrons begin to share frequencies with each other that are above the frequency of thougths. Through this other intuitive abilites such as clairvoyance and precognition are developed. With the exercising of the silent meditation, a pure thought-free clarity of mind can be achieved. If the forehead centre begins to open, a pressure behind the eyebrows is noticeable followed by a pleasant tingling and sparkling. This is where  the first sparks of happiness develope which in the wake rise further up and help to open our gate to heaven, the crown centre.

The area of the forehead centre brings a person in connection with experiences from previous incarnations and we learn to integrate these experiences through the front centre into the consciousness. In conjunction with a pure and warm heart, it is also the centre of intuitive abilities such as clairvoyance and already conveys the cosmic awareness  that everything is connected to everything.

With an open front centre an inner freedom and majesty over the entire mental and emotional range is achieved. If we anchor ourselves in this way, nothing can cut us down.

**Disturbed Function:** The described functions of the frontal centre are rarely or never uncovered in most people. Without spiritual transformation methods – in particular the practicing of the silent meditation – an uncovering and opening of this centre cannot be reached.

## 7. Crown Centre

**Healthy Function:** The crown centre is located at the highest point of our head. In the vibrational octave of visible light, the crown centre corresponds to the colour violet. The physical representation of the crown centre is the pineal gland. In it the electrons can reach the highest possible vibration through the exchange of high-frequency light particles and can thus set the process in motion that has already been described within physics as enlightenment. This state of awareness goes beyond the cosmic consciousness and also opens up access to the hyperspace – to heaven. With enlightenment an important step to regaining all-encompassing immortality is reached. A blazing flame of everlasting happiness is kindled in the open crown centre. The connection to the source of all being in hyperspace is achieved – once and for all. With further development the entire body can be seized by this high-frequency light flame and the complete liberation and freedom of movement are reached, with the possibility of transition into hyperspace – equated with an ascension.

Due to the methods already learnt and applied, we might have felt that these energy centres indeed exist. If we are to realize our full happiness potential, it is important to activate these energy centres in order to let the happiness-flow through our body become stronger. Here, we can through simple means, namely our own hands, cause a higher excitation of our energy centres.

## ACTIVATION OF THE CHAKRAS
## WITH HAND MOVEMENTS

We can effectively radiate and transmit bioplasma through our palms. If we want to activate our chakras, we can support this with the inside of our hands.

**The Exercise Execution:** For this purpose we move our palms a distance of a few inches over the front side of our body at the level of a chakra. We circle our palms over two adjacent chakras – our hands describing a circle here in a diameter of two to four inches. If we perform this exercise for one to two minutes, we may feel a pleasant tingling in the palms of our hands and in the chakras.

Using this, we can activate the centres and form

a vortex of energy. The exercise can be performed on all seven main energy centres.

This method is of course also suitable as a partner exercise by assisting another person to activate their energy system. Whether as an individual or a partner exercise, the action can be performed while standing, sitting or lying down. An exercise period of about one to two minutes is recommended for each of the centres.

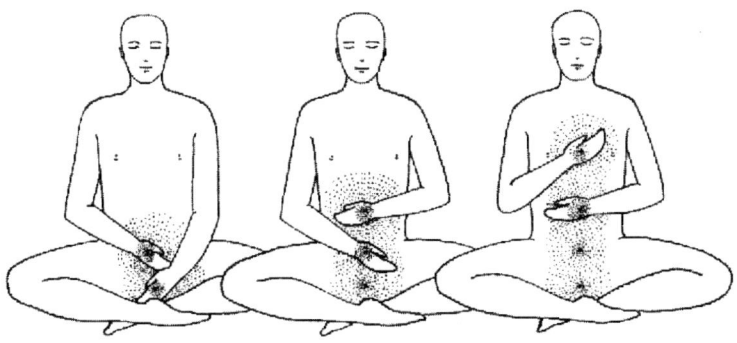

## FROM THE TWO-POINT TO THE ZERO METHOD

As we have learned from the previous chapters to increase the biophotons in our bodies and therefore also helped our consciousness achieve "quantum-jumps", the following quantum healing methods can be used very effectively.

The higher the level of vitality that we have, the stronger our self-healing potential. Especially if we practiced and learnt in the silent meditation to take the position of an uninvolved observer in order to calm the stream of thoughts, we will bring about an energy pooling inside of us. With higher energy density comes better self-healing results.

If we can assume a state of consciousness in which we are free of thoughts as much as possible and the little happiness flame is ignited in our pituitary gland, which then ascends to the apex, we can apply successful methods of quantum healing to ourselves and others.

*The Two-Point Method*

In current literature about quantum healing the two-point method is explained for self-healing treatments. Starting with the feeling of happiness that we can produce by silent meditation, we put one hand or some fingers on a point we want to treat on the body surface and the other hand, or some of it's fingers, to another part of the body. In the healing language this is called the triangulation. We combine the happy flame in our consciousness with the two points that we touch with our hands and as a result an energy flow is created which leads to an increase in the bioplasma-level in the two contact points.

The vibrant biophoton field in our body contains all the information that our body needs to function optimally at each point so it can be healthy. If a position in our body hurts or we get the impression that a body region is not provided well with energy, bioplasma energy is supplied again in this way and the body part can be regulated better. Some symptoms such as headaches and muscle pain, tension and emotional burdens or sickness in the stomach area can be treated easily and successfully with this method.

## The One-Point Method

But there also exists a much easier way. Provided, we have generated a much higher biophoton concentration within ourselves, we can also apply the one-point method. We then place the inner side of the left hand on our heart chakra. With the right hand we touch a body point that we want to treat. This can be a place on our own body or a spot that needs to be treated in another person. Due to the fact that we have put our left hand on the heart chakra, the side-centre in our palm is continuously charged. Indeed, it is very effective to absorb the bioplasma energy directly from a chakra – it is best from the heart chakra, as the chakra is located in the middle of the seven major energy centres.

Through our arms a cycle of bioplasma energy is created, radiating from the heart. We should free ourselves of the self-centered attitude that we have healed something.

What heals us, is the ubiquitous quantum field that is fed from the inexhaustible source of ELI in the hyperspace. And if we connect ourselves through meditation with this quantum field by reducing our stream of thoughts, we are penetrated and charged by this

113

quantum field. In this way we become the channel for the healing forces of the quantum field – a blessing to ourselves and to others.

*The Zero Point Method*

The simplest method of quantum healing is the zero point method, where we do not need to touch any point on our or another body. We just start with our own pure consciousness. If the bioplasma flame in the pituitary gland has already ignited, we imagine that the light and the energy of this flame goes everywhere. Those who cannot feel the flame yet, should focus on their heart chakra, because there is always life energy as long as we live.

We only need to imagine the place where this energy is supposed to flow to and it is already there. If we imagine this place to be the point where we perceive the greatest amount of light and energy in us, then this energy will pass to the place where we would like it to go. Two partners who love each other know this and will have experienced it many times. When they think of their partner, the energy immediately begins to flow more. This pleasant stream gives us the feeling of love – it is biophoton energy.

Depending on our individual spiritual development, there is always a chakra where the energy is strongest. From there we consciously connect with the place that we want to heal. This is the zero point method.

We can also apply this method in conjunction with a symbol. For this we simply contemplate a symbol such as the ELI-icon or the Ancient Word Matrix, while we take on a pure state of consciousness free of thoughts within us. And in our imagination we then connect the symbol with the place that we want to treat.

# 6. NATURAL MEANS OF SUPPORT FOR QUANTUM HEALING

## CRYSTALS AND GEMSTONES

Since ancient times, crystals and gemstones have been a thing of major fascination to us. This is due to their beauty, but also to their rarity. Crystals and gems were used long into the past and in ancient times in order to purify the mind and to gain inner clarity. A pure rock crystal, for example, provides because of its regular shape an orderly and whole ideal state which we are all longing for and aspire to through our spiritual transformation efforts.

The findings of modern physics confirm these purely intuitive feelings that we have when looking at a crystal or a gemstone. This is because we now know that the atoms by which all matter is constructed, are arranged in a regular and organised manner in crystals.

*The Energising Effect*

People who have dealt for a while with gems and crystals and put them on their bodies, especially on the chakras, have experienced that they can augment the energy flow in the body through this. When I first started to use crystals and gemstones 25 years ago, as a tool for spiritual transformation, there was no physical model concept with which their noticeable energising effect could be described.

I found the key to the physical understanding of the energising results of crystalline structures in the findings of modern biophysics. In biological organisms there exist coherent electromagnetic radiation fields – biophotons, which control the chemical metabolic processes in the cells. What does this have to do with crystals?

Quite simply – if light particles in general (the photons), penetrate a crystal, they can be reflected by the regular and parallel layers of arranged atoms within the crystal.

In this case the photons, which can also be considered as waves in quantum physics, are arranged regularly. Before the photons radiate into the crystal, they are usually incoherent, meaning that, their peaks and troughs are not mutually aligned. It is as if one were to observe a moving water surface, for example on the sea or on a lake. The wave pattern is completely chaotic and irregular. Within the crystal, a part of the photons is sorted instead. Similarly to wave crest to wave crest and trough to trough. This creates coherent photons and these will then have the same characteristics as the coherent biophotons in our cells. So, if we put crystalline structures, such as mountain crystals or gemstones on our body, the stones provide us with coherent biophotons and the biophoton concentration can rise inside us.


*The Influence of the Sun*

In the same way, coherent standing waves are formed in crystalline structures with characteristics similar to the coherent biophotons in our cells. The highly ordered photon field in crystals and gemstones can provide us with coherent photons better, the more energy is supplied from the outside to them in the form of incoherent photons. This energy is supplied by the daylight in the visible range of the photons. Our sun supplies us on the earth with all photon frequencies that are needed for life on earth. It is therefore reasonable to not keep crystals and gems – if possible – in the dark, locked away, but to instead let them have as much light as possible, preferably in the form of direct sunlight. In this way a part of the interspersed light energy from the sun is refined by the crystals, that is, converted into coherent photons.

If a crystal or gemstone is exposed over a longer period of time to direct sunlight, the electrons in the crystal atoms are fully programmed to receive and emit these photons again. From some electron models it is known that electrons can save their interactions with photons in their interior in the form of light patterns. This information of the ordered exchange of photons may be transferred by placing it on the body surface of a biological organism. This is the scientific basis of the ancient lithotherapy – the healing with gemstones – which has experienced an enormous boom and a renaissance in recent decades.

## Cleaning of Negative Energy

However, lithotherapy also has its dark sides, which one should be informed about as well. The electrons in the atoms of crystals and gemstones can receive transmitted light patterns that originate from the consciousness of another biological being. Thoughts and feelings also correspond to electromagnetic fields which are established by the electrons between each other. In consequence this means that crystals and gems can record and save negative thoughts and feelings as well.

Therefore, when using crystals and gems, we should neutralise their energy every time, after each laying. This is best done under running water. After an application one can place the crystals and gems on a small plate and put it into a sink, directly under the weak flow from the water tap. If one has the possibility of cleaning the stones in the garden pond under a fountain or in a small stream, should of course prefer this to the tap. After that,  the  stones can be recharged in the sunlight.

If one observes these basic rules of charging and cleaning crystals and gemstones may not only be of lasting value, but also honorable companions of our spiritual transformation.

*Crystal-"Siblings"*

In addition to the necessity to purify crystals and gemstones of mental patterns, there is another effect that sets certain limits to their value for the spiritual transformation. Who ever for example acquires a rock crystal or an amethyst on a gemstone market, never knows where the close "relatives" of this stone have ended up. Such crystals grow mostly in druses, spherical cavities, in which they have developed together with many other crystals from a common dense and hot liquid primary matter. With each other, related crystals can exchange energy patterns over large distances and therefore establish a certain energy equilibrium between all of them, which prevents anyone of the sibling crystals rising above the average enery level. If now some of the sibling crystals are located in places where an energy drain exists, all of the sibling crystals are effectively chained to each other, so that a certain level of energy cannot be exceeded by any of them.

Among other things, I for this reason, for the time being have, turned away since the early 1990's from the use of crystals and gemstones, in order to not get into a situation that would have precluded a further energy increase.

## The Uniqueness of Natural Diamonds

In a certain kind of gems this risk of uncontrolled long-range coupling to low-energy areas, however, does not exist, because each of them is unique and grown under extreme conditions at the highest pressure and the highest temperature in the depths of the earth – here we are now talking about natural diamonds. These always grow as single crystals.

Everyone thinks of diamonds immediately as being expensive and processed into valuable jewelery polished diamonds – the brilliants. A diamond of one carat often costs more than 1,000 euros and therefore such brilliants are not a reccommendation in support of spiritual transformation for everyone. One carat is the weight unit for diamonds and corresponds to 0.2 grams. In addition, brilliants are cut in diagonal angles against the plane of the regular atomic layers and in this way the coherence effects in brilliants keep within limits. The best always comes from nature, and it is the same with diamonds. The uncut natural diamond, as it is hauled from the earth, provides the highest energising potential.

Now everyone will object that larger natural diamonds are not exactly inexpensive either. But they don't have to be large natural diamonds, it will suffice for a grain sized diamond slightly under one millimeter. Such small natural diamonds are hauled in large quantities, but are of no interest to the classic jewelery industry since they are too small to be cut.

With such small natural diamonds the coherence effects described can still be generated and with them, natural diamond products with high carat numbers can be produced relatively inexspensively.

These were the main reasons for me turning back to lithotherapy, but this time exclusively based on the use of natural diamonds. Today, we have a number of very innovative natural diamond products at our disposal which not only fascinate us with their aesthetics because of the artisanal quality of processing, but can also provide a significant contribution to our physical-mental-spiritual integration and to our spiritual transformation because of their strongly energising effect.

In the following section we take a look at the many uses of natural diamonds to vitalise us during relaxation and meditation.

## QUANTUM HEALING WITH NATURAL DIAMOND PRODUCTS

The diamond is the most precious of the precious stones – it is the king of gems, the hardest and purest mineral found in nature. We humans have so far failed to produce harder material synthetically. Due to its chemical nature and its particular physical properties the natural diamond is wonderfully suited to increase in an optimal manner the biophoton concentration in biological organisms.

The natural diamond is composed of a hundred percent carbon, the main component of organic molecules. Our life is based on carbon and therefore, the coherent photon energy of the diamond can perfectly be brought into our bodies, when we just let them come close enough to us.

Using different and independent measuring methods the beneficial effects of natural diamond products on the vitality of humans has been confirmed. So, I have been able to demonstrate myself the increase of the biophoton concentration using the natural diamonds, with a biophysical measuring method. Others have found through the application of the dark field microscopy that by using the influence of natural diamonds the blood-picture improved - clumped red blood cells separated and floated freely again. It was also confirmed by a specialist using a biomedical measurement method that metabolic parameters improved under the influence of a natural diamond product and thus a higher vitality level was reached.

*Dealing with Natural Diamonds*

Methods of quantum healing, such as the ones described in the previous chapter: the two-point-, one-point- and zero-point-method, work even more effectively if natural diamond products are used to strengthen and support the quantum field.

Here, natural diamond products that can be placed directly on or carried on the body are especially well suited. This includes diamond energy discs, which are placed on the chakras or any other part of the body in an application while lying down. For massages and energy work, diamond rods can also be used, which significantly improve effects that can be obtained than with rock crystals.

For support in everyday life and to further increase the vitality and performance, natural diamond jewelery or energy clip products are suited, which can be simply worn on the body or within a pocket.

As already mentioned, there is no need to fear that the untreated natural diamond is coupled to other natural diamonds´ energy. Another advantage of the natural diamond consists of its inherent high vibrations due to its exceptional hardness so that it owns such a high natural frequency, that no negative mental vibration pattern can be stored inside it. It is therefore not necessary to clean natural diamond product´s energy under running water after each use. At the most a cleaning may be required from time to time to eliminate outer build up, which can result from wearing the product on the skin.

Natural diamonds also provide a more effective service to our energy system when they are charged, preferably in sunlight. However, the natural diamond also works when it is worn under clothing next to the skin or even if it is embedded in other opaque materials such as natural cork granules. One should also know that the diamond can store energy rich photons, which can penetrate solid matter, in its atomic lattice-structure.

Such high-energy quanta are omnipresent and the diamond is, like any other solid body, continuously in thermodynamic equilibrium with its quantum environment.

## Chakra Meditation and Diamond Energy Discs

We make ourselves comfortable on a blanket and put a diamond energy disk, which we have previously warmed up with our hands, on a chakra. We can now refuel from the quantum ocean.

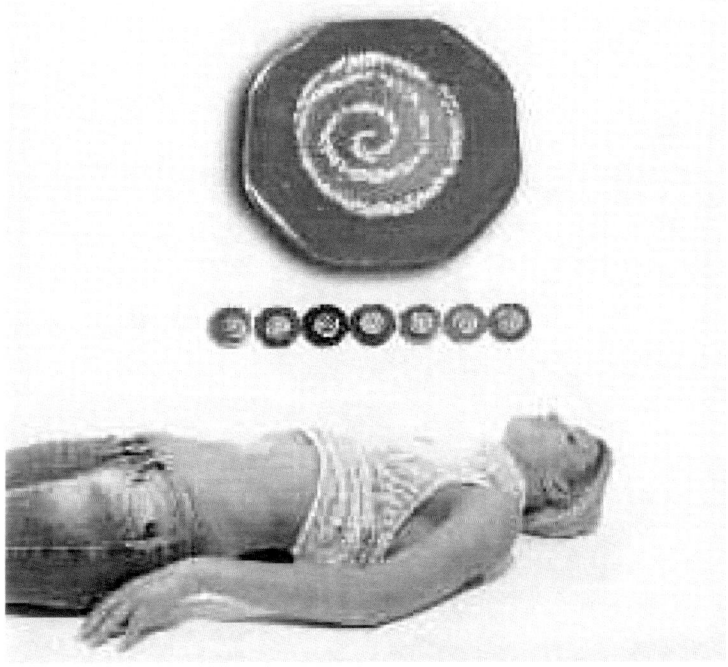

A diamond energy disc (approximately 3 inches in diameter) one carat natural diamond embedded in solid glass.

We can optimise the absorbtion of the coherent photons generated by the natural diamond over the chakras. During the placing of a diamond energy disc, we can apply the same breathing-, relaxing- and silent-meditation methods as described in the previous chapters.

*Chakra-Spinal-Massage with the Diamond Energy Wand*

In a partner exercise one can massage the spine of the other with a diamond energy wand. The person who gets the massage should sit on a stool and try to sit in an upright but relaxed posture. Both the round and the pointed rod of solid glass have a pleasantly soft and smooth surface. The simultaneous use of a good massage oil is recommended. The massaged area to the left and the right of the spine can then be treated with a diamond energy bar. Before the application the masseur goes into a meditative attitude and tries to activate his happy flame. With slight pressure the diamond rod is then passed up and down to the left and right side of the spine by the masseur.

This is a powerful exercise for the basic activation of the chakras. As the illustration on page 102 shows, the chakras develop in a funnel shape from the spine to the body front. An energising massage application around the spine with a diamond energy  bar is therefore set up where the energy vortices of the chakras root are.

The essence electrons in the central nervous

126

system are strongly activated with diamond energy by this chakra spine massage and intensify their information and photon exchange with the body matter surrounding them. The result of such an application can be affected and awaken deep layers of our soul. This method is thus ideally suited for activation before a silent meditation or an introspection.

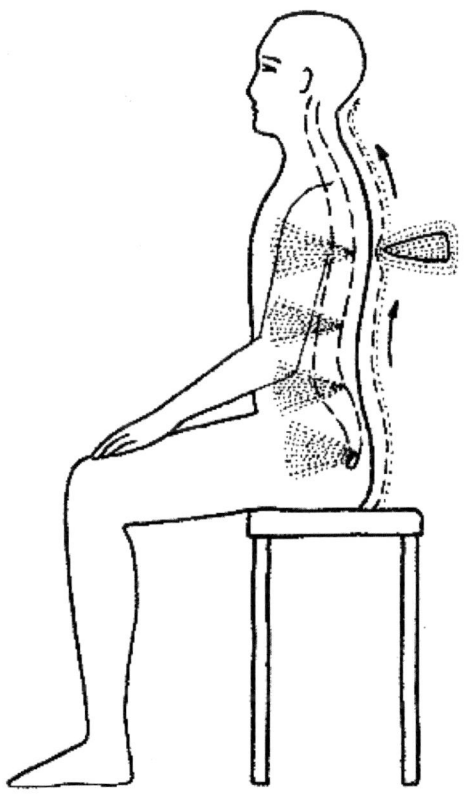

*Chakra-Vertebral-Column-Massage with Diamond Energy Wand*

*Wide Range of Applications*

Of course we can apply both a diamond energy disc as well as the diamond energy wand at any body site where we want the beneficial effect of the diamond to do its quantum work. A massage application with the diamond energy wand can also be done in other places such as strained neck muscles or the hand and foot reflexology.

There are now a number of fascinating natural diamond products with which we can raise our biophoton concentration. In addition to the described diamond energy plates and wands there are also highly concentrated diamond graphite chips and natural diamond jewelry that can be worn in a jacket pocket or directly on the body in order to accompany us in everyday life with their harmonising and energy stregthening effect throughout the day.

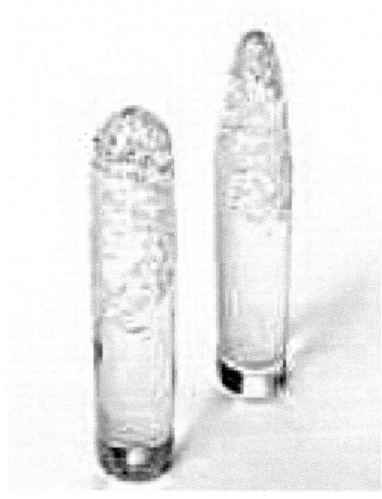

*Diamond Energy Wands (approximately 12 cm length): 1,5 carat natural diamond in solid glass*

Diamond light bodies and glasses can enrich the air in a room or drinks with high biophoton concentration.

The future of lithotherapy therefore belongs to the natural diamond, which with its high vibration properties and its integrity can make a valuable and effective contribution to our spiritual development.


## MEASUREMENTS OF VITALITY AND AWARENESS

The development of particular energy systems can be measured using biophysical methods. A detailed description of the functioning of a measurement method can be found in my book   The Original Word – The Physics of God.  The two recordings on the next page show the energy status of the meridian system on the finger of a test person before and after the charging with a natural diamond product.

The three shots on the page after the next show three differently developed human energy systems using the example of the heart-small-intestine meridian (left little finger). As long as there are energy blocks in a person, the flow of energy remains disturbed. With increasing development of the energy system, the biophoton concentration becomes stronger, until the energy flow eventually becomes perfectly harmonious because the happy flame has started or a blazing flame of bioplasma may even have ignited.

Evaluated bioplasma concentration on the finger of a test person

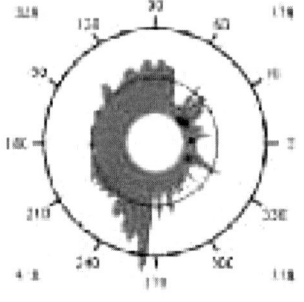

*Prior to contact with a natural diamond product*

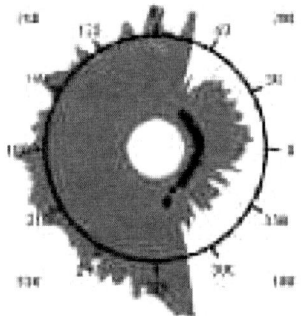

*After contact with a natural diamond product*

Bioplasma concentrations at the terminal point of the
heart-small-intestine meridian (small left finger)

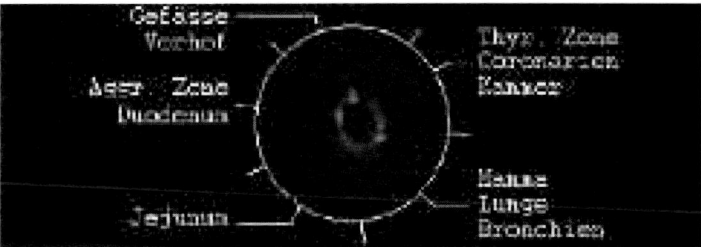

*Weak radiation*

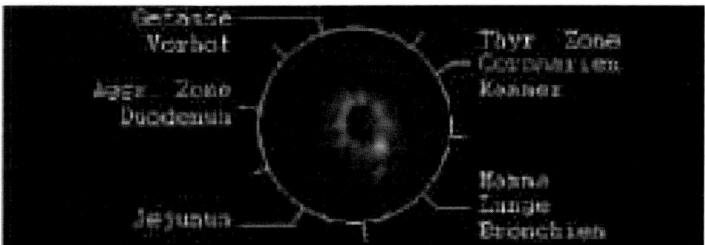

*Average radiation*

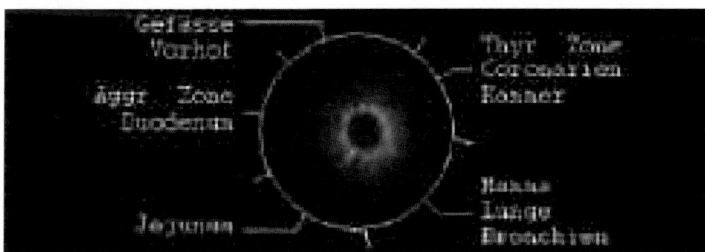

*Strong radiation*

# 7. ABOUT EATING AND DRINKING AND FASTING

When we strive for the development of our happiness potential, inevitably the question of optimal nutrition is asked, which supports us in our spiritual transformation quest.

In order to increase the concentration of biophotons in our body, we need mainly food, which has not been denaturated and processed too much. In our western civilization, the so-called abundance-society, many people are overweight and suffering the consequences of poor nutritional habits. Meat consumption has increased drastically in the period after the Second World War. This results not only in an increase in health problems, but also considerable environmental and ethical issues, for example factory farming.

Anyone, who has ever viewed hens in battery farms or of a pig in a breeding farm and also looks at how these animals are then killed; before their groceries arrive freshly packed in the refrigerated counter of the supermarket, looses the appetite for such food. Some consumer-conscious users then deviate to steaks and roasts from animal friendly farming − but can you kill animals in a human way?

*Our Food conveys Messages as well*

People are so far removed from the production of food that they usually don't worry about the related atrocities. But according to interactions in the laws of physics the information of horror and psychological distress, through which an animal has gone while being killed, is stored in a piece of meat as well, because the electrons of animals also save this information. This is information about repression and death that we take in.

I could very quickly discover the positive impact on my consciousness and my inner spiritual perception, when I switched to a largely vegetarian diet 25 years ago. Dreams became clearer and access to unconscious layers occurred to me noticeably easier. The ability to remember grew. Long past events or experiences from past lives could be remembered more clearly.

In the 1990s I have tried different types of vegetarian diets, each of them over longer periods of time. At first, I gave up only meat, then I stopped eating any eggs and dairy products. Later, I left behind animal products completely − and thus no more honey, no wool and no more leather in clothing − and I nourished myself purely on a vegan diet. I temporarily stopped cooking and found that I could live basically only eating raw plant food.

My raw food experiment lasted about a year until it came to an abrupt end when I bit into a crusty baguette during a vacation in France.

I made my raw food experiment when I was about 40 years old, and after this raw food year my body was clearly rejuvenated, I felt physically as though I was in my early 20s.

Nevertheless, I would not like to give a preference to any of the many variations of the vegetarian diet, but I generally advocate for a form of nutrition that causes as little suffering to other living beings as possible. I can only encourage every spiritual seeker to try all forms of vegetarian diets for a certain period of time to realise the potential that lies in each of them. If one experiments deliberately with it, one recognises, how the body tries at first to remain in the old eating habits that have been the norm for decades, until after a detoxification and purification process they assume a new, higher energy state.

Today, I live largely vegetarian and try to avoid acidification.

*Drinking Water*

In addition to the solid food that we eat, what we

drink is also significant. By this, I mean primarily the drinking water that we use for the preparation of our food and drink.

In many regions, the drinking water that comes out of the tap, though free from germs and bacteria, can contain, depending on the type of public water supply, a variety of harmful pollutants. One should not be deceived by the fact that the concentration of pollutants lies below the legal limit, because who wants to ensure that these limits are actually relevant in the long-term assessment of the harmfulness? In rural areas  high concentrations of nitrate and pesticides in drinking water are often found and in regions that obtain their water by bank filtration of surface waters such as lakes or rivers, there is a veritable cocktail of a variety of dilute chemicals such as medicines and heavy metals found in it.

Apart from these man-made civilization contaminants, public drinking water is often very hard, that is , strongly calcareous. Although, the manufacturers of mineral waters often advertise that high levels of minerals such as calcium and magnesium are so important for our diet – they neglect to mention that we cannot cover our mineral needs of calcium and magnesium through the drinking of mineral waters, but only in the form of suitable foods. If we were to meet our calcium needs  from just mineral water, we would have to drink five to ten litres of mineral water daily, because our body can not absorb these minerals just very well. Instead, one or two bananas would be sufficient to meet the daily calcium requirements.

Drinking water that is too strongly calcareous, is basically saturated. It can hardly support us in detoxifying and cleansing our body, because it is so overloaded that it can no longer dissolve other substances. If you prepare drinks with hard water you notice for example that the flavours of tea do not get into the water. A film forms on the water surface, which also sticks to the inside of the cup in an ugly way when you drink the tea. Nor can such lime water remove the toxins caused by metabolism from our body.

**Reverse Osmosis:** This is what I have drunk, since 1990, if possible, only water which is substantially free of dissolved minerals. To achieve this, I use a water treatment technology, which is known as reverse osmosis. For this purpose, drinking water that comes from the tap, is pressed through a very fine pore membrane that almost only lets the water molecules through and rejects other materials dissolved in the water, such as calcium ions, heavy metals and other pollutants. Such reverse osmosis appliances for the home are now available relatively inexpensively and can be easily integrated as under-table-units in any kitchen sink. As a downstream filter, these devices usually also contain an active carbon filter that improves the taste of the water and additionally binds the last remnants of pollutants.

It is just a widespread fallacy that we can achieve spiritual transformation only through mental training without paying attention to the cleansing and detoxifying our body. A natural diet and pure water that is low on minerals are equally important.

*Supporting the Cleaning Processes*

We should be careful to drink enough, one to two litres every day. Drinking is especially important, if we have resolved an energetic blockage through appropriate methods. On a physical level, the dissolving of such blockages is always connected with the fact that the chemical milieu in the body area concerned is also changing and for this the body wants to excrete certain waste products and pollutants that were bound here.

The cleansing effect of fasting is also known in all spiritual traditions. When we fast, we can rid our bodies of deposits and slags. While fasting, it is especially important to make sure that we drink enough.

If we get sore muscles or headaches after applying a transformation method, we can support the cleaning process by an adequate intake of fluids – of pure water.

*The Reduction of Acidification*

It is important to keep an eye on the body's pH. Optimally, it should be more than seven, so that it is slightly basic. You can control it with test strips from a pharmacy. The best way to determine the body's own pH is by measuring saliva or urine. Many people are chronically too acidic. An acidified organism ages faster because of the many free radicals. Acidification refers to electron deficiency, which leads to a lowering of biophoton concentration and thus also to reduced vitality. Such an electron deficiency can therefore hinder the lighting of the happiness flame. We need a certain amount of electrons, because the electrons are the ones, which exchange the biophotons and thus enable a strong bioplasma concentration.

An acidic body is like a wet piece of wood that cannot be lit and can only smoulder. In this case no spiritual transformation methods will help.

In the condition of hyperacidity, the body should be brought back to a more basic range through an appropriate diet and the supply of basic salts. Also helpful are ionisers for the drinking water, from which alkaline water with an excess of electrons can be generated.

# EPILOGUE

Spiritual transformation and quantum healing have scientific bases. The relationship between the biophoton concentration and vitality and consciousness of a person lies on hand.

In this book effective methods were presented, that anyone can apply for themselves in order to achieve a higher level of vitality and awareness. However, the individual possiblities for consciousness transformation are far from being exhausted with this. Those who follow the path of self-awareness, should be willing to try methods, which are new to them and still unknown.

Also recommended is an intellectual exchange with like-minded people who also want to develop themselves and with whom you can practice such applications. Just as the cells in our body can share information better with each other through a stronger biophoton field, we have to rely on an optimised information exchange in our social development as well.

The more clarity we have created within ourselves, the more clearly we will be able to communicate with other people.

We need more information and more photon exchange in dealing with people. Love is photon exchange, and that is what is lacking the most in our society.

If each of us lights a pure mental candle inside ourselves, then it will not only warm our hearts but it will become bright and clear when dealing with each other. We will all need this light within us to go through the development steps that are now pending and in order to be able to cope with the challenges of this time.


Self-Awareness Seminars on the Topics:

Dr. Michael König organises together with a team of experienced users on a continuous basis the following seminars:

Basic Seminar I:   Introduction to Quantum Practice*
Basic Seminar II:  Training for Quantum Practitioner*
Basic Seminar III: Certification for Quantum

                          Practitioner*

## ABOUT THE AUTHOR

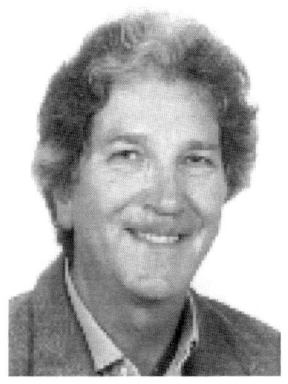

Dr. Michael König, born in 1957, is a quantum physicist and has been dedicated for nearly 30 years to the exploration of the relationship between mind and matter. Between 1987 and 2004 he directed a private research institute and obtained patents in the field of complimentary medicine. As one of the pioneers of the New Physics and of the Shift of Paradigms, he is a sought for referent and lecturer at international conferences, universities and in documentaries. For many years he has also organised spiritual workshops.

Interesting Links:
www.drmichaelkoenig.de
www.NaturdiamantShop.de

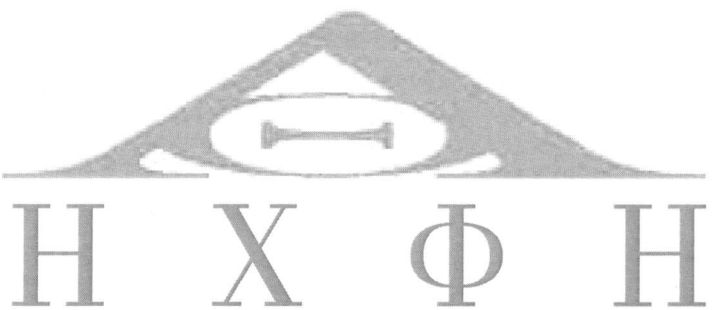